THE

DASH
DIET
Action Plan

THE
DASH
DIET
Action Plan

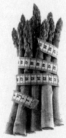

PROVEN TO LOWER
BLOOD PRESSURE
AND CHOLESTEROL
WITHOUT MEDICATION

Marla Heller, MS, RD

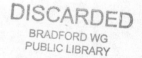
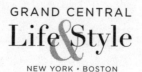

GRAND CENTRAL
Life&Style
NEW YORK · BOSTON

The nutrition advice in this book is based on the DASH diet, developed in the National Institutes of Health studies. It is not intended to replace advice or treatment provided by your physician. Please consult with your physician before making any dietary changes. The author disclaims any liability arising directly or indirectly from The DASH Diet Action Plan.

Nutritional analyses on the menus in this book were obtained using Nutritionist Pro, First DataBank.

Grand Central Life & Style
Hachette Book Group
237 Park Avenue
New York, NY 10017

www.HachetteBookGroup.com

Grand Central Life & Style is an imprint of Grand Central Publishing.
The Grand Central Life & Style name and logo are trademarks of Hachette Book Group, Inc.

The Hachette Speakers Bureau provides a wide range of authors for speaking events. To find out more, go to www.hachettespeakersbureau.com or call (866) 376-6591.

Printed in the United States of America

First Life & Style Edition: September 2011
10 9 8

Library of Congress Control Number: 2011933985

To my husband, Richard

CONTENTS

THE
DASH
DIET
Action Plan

CHAPTER 1

CONQUERING HYPERTENSION AND HEART DISEASE

When you were a child, your grandmother probably told you to drink your milk, eat your fruits and vegetables, and go outside and play. This is still great advice, and shows that our fundamental ideas of good nutrition hold up over time.

The Dietary Approaches to Stop Hypertension diet—better known as the DASH diet—is a "new" healthy eating plan that has been proven to help reduce blood pressure and cholesterol. It is based on the same great advice that our grandmothers' generation lived by—which, somehow, Americans seem to have forgotten. The DASH diet is grounded in healthy eating principles that, in addition to lowering blood pressure, are associated with lower risk of heart disease, stroke, and cancer. It can support reaching and maintaining a healthy weight. No conflicting information, no magic combinations, no forbidden foods—just fabulous healthy eating.

The 2010 Dietary Guidelines for Americans recommend the DASH eating plan for everyone. And, the DASH diet formed the basis for MyPlate dietary guidelines from the USDA.

When you follow the DASH Diet Action Plan, you will eat lots of fruits and vegetables, combined with low-fat dairy foods, lean meat, poultry, fish, some nuts and beans, and grains. The plan is low in saturated fat and cholesterol; has a moderate amount of protein; and is rich in vitamins, minerals, and fiber.

Understanding Blood Pressure

More than sixty-eight million Americans have high blood pressure and another seventy million have prehypertension. It is the leading cause of heart attacks and strokes. If your blood pressure goes too low you may feel lightheaded. If it goes too high there might not be any symptoms, or it could trigger a stroke. If blood pressure remains high, it can lead to congestive heart failure, kidney failure, hardening of the arteries, stroke, and other complications.

What is a diet?

A diet is not just a plan for losing weight; a diet refers to the way we eat. Any eating pattern is a diet.

You might not have learned that you had high blood pressure until your physician detected it in a routine physical exam. You probably had no symptoms. You may not be able to detect that your blood pressure is high unless you check it on a regular basis. Since you often don't feel that anything is wrong, you might not keep it as well controlled as your physician would like. This is one of the reasons hypertension has been called the "silent killer."

Blood pressure is composed of two numbers. Systolic is the "top" number and diastolic is the "bottom" number. If your blood pressure is 120 over 80, the 120 is the systolic pressure and

80 is the diastolic. Blood pressure is considered to be high (hypertension) if the systolic is higher than 140 or if the diastolic is more than 90. (Your physician might consider you to have high blood pressure at slightly lower numbers if there are other medical complications to consider.)

Blood Pressure Definitions

Normal: Systolic 90-119 and diastolic 60-79.

Prehypertension: Systolic 120-139 and/or diastolic 80-89.

Stage I Hypertension: Systolic 140-159 and/or diastolic 90-99.

Stage II Hypertension: Systolic 160 or higher and/or diastolic 100 or greater.

A new category of "prehypertension" has been identified as systolic blood pressure between 120 and 139, or diastolic between 80 and 89. When blood pressure is high, it forces the heart to beat harder to move the blood and can cause premature hardening or other damage to the arteries.

High blood pressure is not an equal opportunity disease. Men are at higher risk of complications than women with the same blood pressure. African Americans and older people are also at higher risk than other ethnic groups and younger people with the same blood pressure readings. This makes it even more important to control hypertension.

Blood pressure can be high for unknown reasons, which is called "essential hypertension." It can also be elevated due to another disease process, such as overproduction of certain hormones or kidney disease. This is called "secondary hypertension" since it occurs secondary to another disease.

Why DASH?

Research sponsored by the National Institutes of Health (NIH) has shown that this healthy diet can lower blood pressure as well as medication. Results are quick, with many people seeing lower blood pressure in only fourteen days with the DASH diet. Adding weight loss (when needed), exercise, and other healthy lifestyle choices further improve the blood pressure benefits. Why does the DASH diet make such a difference? And how does it differ from the average American diet?

A diet that is rich in minerals, high in fiber, and low in saturated fat can help lower blood pressure. Many of the beneficial nutrients are found in fruits and vegetables, along with low-fat dairy foods—all of which are deficient in the typical American diet.

The old food guide pyramid (developed by the USDA and the U.S. Department of Health and Human Services) recommended having two to four fruits and three to five vegetables each day. The DASH diet recommends four to five fruits and four to five vegetable servings each day. The DASH diet is now recommended in the 2010 Dietary Guidelines for Americans and MyPlate (the new USDA food guide). Translated into standard measures by MyPlate, the recommended DASH consumption is two cups of fruit and two-and-a-half cups of vegetables. This may seem especially daunting when you realize that only about half of us have even one-half cup of fruit or fruit juice each day. And, frequent meals away from home make it even less likely that we will include enough fruits and vegetables in our meals. Is the DASH plan something that you can incorporate in real life, with many meals eaten in restaurants or fast food places, and with little time for exercise? This book will help you with creative ideas to boost the health quotient of your daily routine, even if you are always on the run.

The DASH Diet Action Plan will help you choose healthy foods and take other actions to aid in the management of your blood pressure and generally improve your health. Will it help you eliminate or reduce the need for blood pressure medication?

Only your doctor can answer that question. Will it help you become healthier? Yes, that it can do. We know that people who follow a diet low in saturated fat and rich in fruits, vegetables, legumes, and other plant protein foods have reduced risk of heart disease and cancer. Exercise, smoking cessation, and no more than moderate consumption of alcohol can provide additional health benefits. You have much to gain from choosing to follow the DASH eating plan.

Why not just take a supplement? If we could find out what the key components were, it seems that it would be much easier to just pop a pill. However, scientific studies attempting to use supplements to control blood pressure have mostly failed. There is something in the mix of nutrients and other food components of the DASH diet that appears to be protective against many diseases. This will be covered later in this book, especially in the chapter discussing the effects of sodium and other minerals on blood pressure.

At the heart of this book is a model menu plan that will show you how to put the DASH diet into effect. It will give you concrete examples of how you can add more fruits and vegetables to your diet, even if many of your meals are eaten away from home or if you are a picky eater. The menu plan in this book is full of fabulous meals, and dashes the belief that everything that tastes great is bad for you. You will find ways to add many foods that you thought would not be allowed in a healthy diet. If a healthy eating plan doesn't include your favorites, chances are you will not be able to follow it for very long.

DASH and More

Weight loss is often a critical component of controlling blood pressure and reducing other health risks. The DASH Diet Action Plan makes it easy to lose weight, since many of the DASH diet foods are more filling than the empty calorie foods that many people over-consume. You will learn how to determine your healthy weight and how to adapt the DASH diet to meet your calorie needs. The satisfying meal plans in this book will make it easier than you think to lose weight. Exercise is another challenge in our over-scheduled lives. A commitment to your health can be sustained with the easy-to-follow tips presented in this book.

Eat Well, Feel Great, Be Healthy

The DASH Diet Action Plan suggests a way of eating and living that you will want to continue. It will give you more energy and help you avoid the negative feelings that come from overeating foods that are high in calories but aren't so rich in nutrients. Exercise will rid you of the sluggish feeling that goes with a "couch potato" lifestyle. You will find ways to customize the plan for your own personal tastes, to make it something that you can really live with.

Many people with high blood pressure have other medical conditions, including heart disease. Fortunately, the DASH diet will also benefit many of these other conditions. Since it is high in fiber and rich in vitamins and minerals, it can help lower cholesterol, may make it easier to control blood sugar, and may reduce the risk of certain types of cancer.

Many of the risk factors for heart disease can be reduced by making diet and lifestyle changes. You can quit smoking, control blood pressure, lower your cholesterol, lose weight, and become more active. And diet may help reduce newly identified risk factors for heart disease, such as homocysteine and C-reactive protein (a marker of inflammation).

Take Action

Now is the time to open your mind about the possibility of improving your health, by choosing to include more fruits and vegetables, other healthy foods, and exercise in your day. This isn't the traditional diet message that focuses on the "bad foods" that should be eliminated from your diet. This is a positive message about adding great healthy foods to give you a pay off in improved blood pressure control and improved health.

Buying this book was your first step. The chapters will provide you with many tools to reach your goals. Menu plans let you translate the DASH diet into action. Adding exercise, weight control, and other lifestyle changes will maximize the benefits. For people who want to understand more about healthy foods, there is a chapter highlighting healthy carbs, fats, and protein-rich foods. For the vegetable-phobic, we will coax you into expanding your diet with new choices. A kitchen makeover will help set the stage for success.

Heart Disease Risk Factors

Controllable:
Cigarette Smoking
Hypertension
High Cholesterol
Low HDL (good cholesterol)
Obesity
Diabetes
Sedentary Lifestyle

Not Controllable:
Family history of early heart disease.
Age 45+ for men and 55+ for women.

Additional Risk Factors:
High homocysteine
High C-reactive protein

Get ready to enjoy healthy eating and a healthy lifestyle, while reaping the rewards in feeling great!

DASHboard

1. Your grandmother told you to drink your milk, eat your fruits and vegetables, and go outside and play. It is still valuable nutrition advice.

2. Over 65 million Americans have high blood pressure, and another 45 million have "prehypertension."

3. Even moderately high blood pressure is linked to increased risk of stroke, heart disease, heart failure, and kidney failure.

4. A diet rich in fruits, vegetables, and low-fat dairy foods can help you lower your blood pressure in 14 days.

5. Exercise, smoking cessation, moderate alcohol consumption, and weight loss can further support lowering blood pressure.

Tracking my Personal DASH Diet Action Plan

	Current	Target
Blood pressure:	_____	_____
Cholesterol:	_____	_____
LDL:	_____	_____
HDL:	_____	_____
Triglycerides:	_____	_____

Additional health goals: _____

_____

_____

_____

_____

_____

CHAPTER 2

YOUR PERSONAL
DASH DIET DESIGN

A typical day's DASH menu at 2,000 calories looks like a decadent feast. When you approach a new diet by focusing on the foods you include, rather than on exclusions, it becomes pleasurable and fun. The following typical day provides a great example.

Breakfast
Freshly Squeezed Orange Juice
Wheaties® with Skim Milk topped with Ripe Raspberries
Cinnamon Raisin English Muffin with a Schmear of Light Cream Cheese

Lunch
Turkey and Light Swiss Cheese on Whole Wheat, smothered with Cranberry Sauce, topped with Romaine Lettuce Leaves

Minestrone Soup
Coleslaw

Snack

Nectarine
Handful of Almonds

Dinner

Italian Bread dipped in Olive Oil
Grilled Salmon with Barbecue Sauce
New Petite Red Potatoes
Haricots Verts dusted with Crushed Hazelnuts
Hearts of Romaine Lettuce spiked with Grape
Tomatoes, Olive Oil Vinaigrette
Very Berry Sundae (Strawberries, Blueberries,
and Blackberries on Light Vanilla Frozen
Yogurt)

What are the easy-to-make changes that boosted the DASH foods in this diet? Fruit was added to make a sweet topping for cereal, a refreshing afternoon snack, and a luscious dessert at dinnertime. Lunch packed in two vegetable servings with a vegetable-stuffed soup and crisp coleslaw. The dinner plate includes potatoes, the very thin French green beans known as *haricots verts*, and a green and red salad. Light dairy foods show up at breakfast, on the lunchtime sandwich, and to make a satisfying sundae for dessert at dinner. Unexpected "real food" toppings include regular salad dressing at dinner, olive oil for the Italian bread, mayonnaise on the coleslaw, tangy cranberry sauce to spice up the all too familiar turkey sandwich, a handful of almonds for a snack, and crushed hazelnuts sprinkled on the green beans.

In this section I will show you how to make the DASH diet work for you. You will learn how many servings add up to the right calories for your needs. You will get specific tips to make the process more intuitive. Complementing this overview are 28 days of meal plans in Chapter 3, tips for staying on track while including restaurant meals in Chapter 4, and weight loss support in Chapter 5. Whether you want to cook most of your meals or eat away from home, you can DASH with ease.

This book will help make following the DASH diet as simple as adding key foods, choosing light and lean, and managing portions.

Dash for Your Calories

In Chapter 5 you will learn how to calculate your calorie needs, if you don't already know where you should be. The following table shows you how to find the DASH diet food plan that matches your personal calorie needs.

Unfortunately, many women, especially if they are short, need to be on a 1,200 to 1,600 calorie plan in order to lose weight. To give more flexibility for the lower calorie ranges, I have reduced the DASH portion sizes for fruits. This way you can include more servings of fruit (just slightly smaller). Usually a diet with more variety will make it easier to include the key DASH nutrients. And variety makes it easier to stay on a plan.

DASH Tips for Intuitive Eaters

This section will give you quick tips to help you make specific changes in your diet so you can reap all the benefits of the DASH diet, without having to think too much about the specifics. For complete meal plans, see Chapter 3. For more tips on restaurant meals, see Chapter 4.

1. **Double up**. The easiest way to be sure to get enough of the key DASH foods is to double up. (This is especially good advice if you tend to overeat, since it has you filling up on the best foods.) Instead of one eight-ounce glass of milk at breakfast, make it a sixteen-ounce glass, and you will have consumed two servings of dairy. One cup of

vegetables makes two servings. One cup of green beans, one small salad, and one cup of potatoes gives you five servings of vegetables at one meal.

2. **Don't double up.** (Sorry for the conflicting advice, there is something here for all sides of your personality.) Watch portion sizes where the calories may mount up quickly and where the foods aren't filling. Juices are one food item you don't want to double up. A large glass of juice has 240 calories, little fiber, and won't keep you feeling full for very long. Limit juice to one serving per day. A DASH serving of juice is six ounces. Get the rest of your fruits and vegetables from whole foods, and you will stay full longer and find it easier to reach and maintain your healthy weight.

3. **Seek out DASH foods.** It's almost like a treasure hunt. Scan menus to find the DASH foods. When you go out to lunch or dinner, keep thinking, "How can I add extra fruits or vegetables?" Add a serving of steamed vegetables to dinners and lunches. Choose to have your pasta sauce on vegetables rather than on pasta. Choose the diced fruit that is often offered as a French fry substitute. Add a salad if the restaurant is vegetable-challenged. At the very least you can add a glass of skim milk.

4. **Stockpile.** Keep your refrigerator and freezer stocked with DASH delights. Buy several bags of frozen vegetables at one time. Keep them fresh after opening by using a clip-tight seal. Buy small portions of cut up fruit from the salad bar. If you buy only what you will eat within one or two days, salad bars can help you avoid waste.

5. **Can you find the hidden DASH foods?** Bring your sandwich to work, and top with grated carrots, shredded red cabbage, and sliced cucumber. Hide a glass of skim milk in your latte or chai tea. Make your own pureed vegetable soup, take a thermos to work, and drink your veggies.

DASH Diet Calorie Adjustments

	1,200	1,600	2,000	2,400
Fruits				
4 oz. servings	3-4	4 - 5		
6 oz. servings			4 - 5	4 - 5
Vegetables	3 - 4	4 - 5	4 - 5	5 or more
Low-fat and nonfat dairy	2 - 3	3	3	3 - 4
Beans and nuts	3 - 4 per week	3 - 4 per week	4 - 5 per week	5 per week
Lean meats, fish, poultry	5 oz.	5 oz.	7 oz.	9 oz.
Whole grains	3	3	3	3 - 5
Refined grains	0	3	5 - 6	6 - 8
Fats and sweets	2	3	4	5

6. **Buy convenience foods that just happen to be healthy foods.** We all are familiar with bagged salad mixes, but how about bagged carrot slices, broccoli, or cauliflower tops, or broccoli slaw (also known as confetti slaw)? Yogurt smoothies without added sugar or skim milk in chuggable bottles make refreshing health drinks.

7. **Keep fresh foods fresh.** Use the new plastic bags that keep foods fresher longer. You are more likely to buy fruits and vegetables if you don't have to worry about them deteriorating before you have a chance to use them.

DASH Diet Servings Check Off Form

Food Groups	Monday	Tuesday	Wednesday	Thursday	Friday	Saturday	Sunday
Grains, starches, sweets — 1 slice bread; 1/3 cup cooked pasta, rice; ½ cup cooked cereal, corn, potatoes; ¼ bagel; 1 oz dry cereal; ½ English muffin, bun; 2 cups popcorn; 2 small cookies	☐☐☐☐☐ ☐☐☐☐☐ ☐☐	☐☐☐☐☐ ☐☐☐☐☐ ☐☐	☐☐☐☐☐ ☐☐☐☐☐ ☐☐	☐☐☐☐☐ ☐☐☐☐☐ ☐☐	☐☐☐☐☐ ☐☐☐☐☐ ☐☐	☐☐☐☐☐ ☐☐☐☐☐ ☐☐	☐☐☐☐☐ ☐☐☐☐☐ ☐☐
Fruits — 4 oz juice, small fruit, ¼ cup dried fruit, ½ cup canned fruit, 1 cup diced raw fruit	☐☐☐☐☐	☐☐☐☐☐	☐☐☐☐☐	☐☐☐☐☐	☐☐☐☐☐	☐☐☐☐☐	☐☐☐☐☐
Vegetables — ½ cup cooked vegetables, 1 cup leafy greens, 6 oz vegetable juice	☐☐☐☐☐	☐☐☐☐☐	☐☐☐☐☐	☐☐☐☐☐	☐☐☐☐☐	☐☐☐☐☐	☐☐☐☐☐
Low fat & nonfat dairy — 8 oz milk, 8 oz , 1 oz reduced-fat cheese, ½ cup cottage cheese	☐☐☐☐☐	☐☐☐☐☐	☐☐☐☐☐	☐☐☐☐☐	☐☐☐☐☐	☐☐☐☐☐	☐☐☐☐☐
Beans, nuts, seeds — ¼ cup beans, nuts, seeds, 2 T peanut butter	☐☐☐☐	☐☐☐☐	☐☐☐☐	☐☐☐☐	☐☐☐☐	☐☐☐☐	☐☐☐☐
Lean meat, fish, poultry, eggs, soy meat substitutes — Each ☐ = 1 oz; 1 egg = 1 oz, 2 egg whites = 1 oz	☐☐☐☐☐ ☐☐☐☐☐	☐☐☐☐☐ ☐☐☐☐☐	☐☐☐☐☐ ☐☐☐☐☐	☐☐☐☐☐ ☐☐☐☐☐	☐☐☐☐☐ ☐☐☐☐☐	☐☐☐☐☐ ☐☐☐☐☐	☐☐☐☐☐ ☐☐☐☐☐
Fats, fatty sauces — 1 T salad dressing; 1 t butter, oil	☐☐☐☐☐	☐☐☐☐☐	☐☐☐☐☐	☐☐☐☐☐	☐☐☐☐☐	☐☐☐☐☐	☐☐☐☐☐
Water, liquids — 8 oz	☐☐☐☐ ☐☐☐☐	☐☐☐☐ ☐☐☐☐	☐☐☐☐ ☐☐☐☐	☐☐☐☐ ☐☐☐☐	☐☐☐☐ ☐☐☐☐	☐☐☐☐ ☐☐☐☐	☐☐☐☐ ☐☐☐☐
Alcohol — 1 oz liquor, 4 ½ oz wine, 12 oz beer	☐☐	☐☐	☐☐	☐☐	☐☐	☐☐	☐☐
Exercise (each ☐ = 10 minutes)	☐☐☐☐ ☐☐☐☐	☐☐☐☐ ☐☐☐☐	☐☐☐☐ ☐☐☐☐	☐☐☐☐ ☐☐☐☐	☐☐☐☐ ☐☐☐☐	☐☐☐☐ ☐☐☐☐	☐☐☐☐ ☐☐☐☐

Grains, starches ——— Vegetables ——— Dairy ——— Fats ———

Fruits ——— Beans, nuts ——— Lean meats ——— Fluid ———

Alcohol ——— Exercise ———

DASHboard

1. Double up on low-cal DASH when you have the chance, especially non-starchy vegetables and low-fat or nonfat dairy.
2. Limit portion sizes on higher calorie foods.
3. Stock your cupboards and fridge with the key DASH diet foods.
4. Sneak in extra DASH foods. Toss extra raw veggies in your sandwich or have a latte with 8 oz. skim milk.
5. Buy DASH convenience foods, such as bagged pre-cut veggies, yogurt smoothies, and single-serve bottles of milk.

Keeping Track

Especially at the beginning, most of us need to keep track of our servings, to see if we are really meeting the DASH diet guidelines. On the preceeding page is an example of a DASH diet tracking form, which can help keep you focused. Mark your goal for the number of servings of each food group (from page 25, in the DASH Calorie Adjustments chart) on the bottom, and then check off each serving you consume during the day. This will show your progress in reaching your goals. You can find larger, downloadable versions of this form on our Website: http://DASHdiet.org/forms.asp.

Tracking my Personal DASH Diet Action Plan

Specific changes I will make in my diet include:

_____

_____

_____

I will track my intake by using:

_____, _____ days per week.

CHAPTER 3

28 DAYS OF DASH MENUS

This chapter provides you with 28 days of menus for a 2,000-calorie daily diet, with adjustments for 1,200 and 1,600 calories. If your calorie needs are different, use the guidelines in Chapter 2 to find out how to reduce (or increase) the calories as needed. Chapter 5 provides information on how to calculate your calorie needs, which is especially important if you are trying to lose weight.

This chapter provides a variety of meal plans, with options for many different eating styles. There are some "grab and go" breakfasts for people who are eating on the run, some vegetarian meals, some meals that are fun indulgences, and meals that you might find in restaurants. You will find many options to accommodate the DASH diet to your lifestyle and preferences. You do not have to follow the meal plans day-by-day, you can choose the days that accommodate your tastes, preferences, and lifestyle.

Where appropriate, serving sizes refer to cooked portions, all weight measures are noted as ounces (oz.), and liquid measures are noted as fluid ounces (fl. oz.), teaspoon (t), tablespoon (T), and cup (c). For example six ounces of strawberries will be more than a cup (depending on the size and whether they are sliced), while six fluid ounces of orange juice is the volume you would get using a measuring cup. I recommend using a digital kitchen scale to help you get the idea of DASH diet serving sizes (and to help with managing calories).

Many of the menus include recipes that are located in Chapter 14. These recipes are indicated by italics, followed by an asterisk, as in *Chicken Cacciatore**.

These menus meet or exceed the nutrition requirements for the DASH diet. The menus were designed to provide 2,000 calories a day, with less than 30% of calories from fat, less than 7% saturated fat, less than 200 milligrams cholesterol, at least 25 grams of fiber, less than 1,750 milligrams of sodium, greater than 4,000 milligrams of potassium, greater than 1,200 milligrams of calcium, and greater than 400 milligrams of magnesium. The diet plan meets or exceeds all other Recommended Dietary Allowance (RDA) values for vitamins and minerals for people over the age of fifty.

The following meal plans have adjustments for 1,200- and 1,600-calorie diets. Any needed adjustments for 1,200 calories are in parentheses, and any 1,600-calorie modifications are in brackets. For example, on the first day's menu plan, someone following a 1,200- calorie plan would have 1 oz. Wheaties with 4 oz. strawberries, 4 oz. juice, and 8 oz. skim milk. The 1,600-calorie plan would include all of the above plus toast and jam. In general, the lower calorie plans have 4 oz. serving sizes of fruits (small versus medium), 1 tablespoon of regular salad dressings, 1 tablespoon of nuts, 0.6 oz. of cheese, and 2 oz. of meat, fish. or poultry at lunch and 3 oz. at dinner. Usually the 1,200-calorie diet is limited in desserts (sigh . . .).

You can make substitutions within food groups for any of these meal plans, to accommodate your taste preferences. When substituting for fruits or vegetables, try to choose other fruits and vegetables that are also rich in potassium. You can find a table of potassium-rich foods in Chapter 10. In order to stay within your calorie guidelines, try not to substitute starchy vegetables (such as potatoes or winter squash) for non-starchy vegetables. Always choose lean meats, fish, or poultry and low fat or nonfat dairy instead of making higher fat substitutions. And avoid higher salt choices.

Week 1

Week 1 Monday 2,000 [1,600] (1,200) Calories

Breakfast

Cereal, Strawberries, Juice, Toast, Milk

1 oz. Wheaties®, topped with 6 oz. strawberries [(4 oz.)]

6 fl. oz. orange juice [(4 fl. oz.)]

1 slice whole wheat toast (0), with 2 t strawberry jam (0)

8 fl. oz. nonfat (skim) milk

Lunch

Half Tuna Sandwich, Side Salad, Nectarine, Milk

half tuna sandwich: 1 slice wheat berry bread (0), with ½ c *low sodium, light tuna salad** [(1/3 c)], topped with ¼ c cucumber slices

side salad: 1 c romaine lettuce, with 8 grape tomatoes, and 2 T nonfat Italian dressing, with no added salt

8 fl. oz. nonfat milk

1 medium nectarine [(small)]

Snack

Almonds and Yogurt

¼ c almonds [(1 T)]

6 oz. nonfat, artificially sweetened, peach yogurt

Dinner

Chicken Piccata, Potatoes, Haricots Verts, Green Salad, Chocolate Chip Cookies, Grapes

3 oz. *Chicken Piccata**

1 serving *Parmesan Potatoes** (0)

½ c haricots verts (skinny French green beans)

green salad: 1½ c mixed greens, topped with 2 T oil and vinegar dressing [(1 T)]

2 chocolate chip cookies [(0)]

1 c grapes (0)

DASH servings: 3 whole grains, 4 fruits, 5 vegetables, 3 dairy, 1 nuts, 6 oz. meats

30

Week 1 Tuesday 2,000 [1,600] (1,200) Calories

Breakfast

Omelet, Toast, Mixed Berries, Juice, Latte

Southwestern Egg White Omelet*

2 slices whole wheat toast [1] (0), topped with 4 t raspberry jam
    [2 t] (0)

1 c mixed blueberries, strawberries, and raspberries

6 oz. peach nectar [(4 fl. oz.)]

coffee latte: 8 fl. oz. nonfat milk and 2 fl. oz. espresso

Lunch

Ham and Swiss Sandwich, Raw Veggies, Apple

ham and Swiss sandwich: 2 slices whole grain bread [(1)], 2 oz. ham,
    and 1 oz. low-sodium, low-fat Swiss cheese [(0.6 oz.)], topped
    with ¼ c shredded cabbage, 2 slices tomato, and mustard

½ c carrot "chips" (crinkle-cut raw carrot chips)

8 grape tomatoes

1 medium Granny Smith apple [(small)]

Snack

Hazelnuts, Cantaloupe, Yogurt

¼ c hazelnuts [(1 T)]

4 oz. cantaloupe

6 oz. nonfat, artificially sweetened strawberry-kiwi yogurt

Dinner

Salmon on a Bed of Mashed Sweet Potatoes, with Broccoli, Mesclun
    Salad, Bread, Frozen Yogurt

4 oz. grilled salmon [(3 oz.)]

½ c mashed sweet potatoes

1 c steamed broccoli

mesclun salad: 1½ c mixed baby greens, topped with 2 T Champaign
    vinaigrette dressing [(1 T)]

1 slice Italian bread (0)

½ c nonfat, artificially sweetened frozen yogurt

DASH servings: 4 whole grains, 3 dairy, 4 fruits, 5+ vegetables, 1 nuts, 8 oz.
meats

Week 1 Wednesday 2,000 [1,600] (1,200) Calories

Breakfast

French Toast Topped with Sliced Canned Peaches, Strawberry-
Banana Smoothie

2 slices whole wheat French toast [(1)], topped with ½ c sliced
peaches [(¼ c)]

smoothie: 4 oz. strawberries, ½ banana, and 8 fl. oz. nonfat milk

Lunch

Open Face Tuna Melt, Oven Fries, Coleslaw, Peas and Carrots, Milk,
Apple

open face tuna melt: ½ c *low sodium tuna salad** [(1/3 c)], with
1 oz. low-sodium, low-fat cheddar cheese [(0.6 oz.)], on 1 slice
whole wheat bread

1 serving *Oven Potato Fries** (½ serving)

1 c coleslaw [(½ c)]

½ c steamed peas and carrots

8 fl. oz. nonfat milk

1 medium Fuji apple [(small)]

Snack

Baby Carrots dipped in Spreadable Cheese, Almonds

8 baby carrots dipped in 1 Light Laughing Cow™ Spreadable Cheese

¼ c almonds [(1 T)]

Dinner

Pollo alla Griglia on a Bed of Mixed Baby Greens, Grape Tomatoes,
and Roasted Potatoes, with Steamed Spinach, Mixed Berries and
Plums

*Pollo alla Griglia** on a bed of 1½ c mixed baby greens, 8 grape tomatoes, ½ c roasted potatoes, and 2 T oil and vinegar dressing [(1 T)]

½ c steamed spinach

1 c mixed raspberries, sliced plums, and blueberries [(½ c)]

DASH servings: 3 whole grains, 4 fruits, 6 vegetables, 3 dairy, 1 nuts, 6 oz.
meats

Week 1 Thursday 2,000 [1,600] (1,200) Calories

Breakfast

Quick Scramblers, Sliced Strawberries, Toast, Juice, Milk

quick scramblers: In microwave-safe dish, sprayed with nonstick cooking spray, microwave ½ c Egg Beaters™ Southwestern Style [(¼ c)], 2 minutes on high.

6 oz. sliced strawberries [(4 oz.)]

1 slice whole wheat toast (0), topped with 2 t strawberry preserves (0)

6 fl. oz. orange juice [(4 fl. oz.)]

8 fl. oz. nonfat milk

Lunch

Beef and Swiss Sandwich, Potato Chips, Grape Tomatoes, Milk, Pluot

lean beef and Swiss sandwich: 2 slices whole wheat bread [(1)], 2 oz. lean beef, 1 oz. low-sodium, low-fat Swiss cheese [(0.6 oz.)], topped with ¼ c shredded romaine lettuce, 2 slices of tomato, and mustard

1 oz. lightly salted baked potato chips [(0)]

8 grape tomatoes

8 fl. oz. nonfat milk

1 pluot (a delicious cross between a plum and an apricot)

Snack

Apple Slices Dipped in Peanut Butter

apple slices from 1 medium apple [(small)], dipped in 2 T natural peanut butter [(1 T)]

Dinner

Lean, Meaty Spaghetti, Green Beans, Dinner Salad, Frozen Yogurt

spaghetti with extra lean meat sauce: 1 c *Lean, Meaty Spaghetti Sauce** on 1 c spaghetti [(½ c)]

½ c green beans

dinner salad: 1½ c green salad, topped with 2 T nonfat Italian dressing, with no added salt

½ c nonfat, artificially sweetened frozen yogurt (0)

DASH servings: 3 whole grains, 4 fruits, 5 vegetables, 3+ dairy, 1 nuts, 7 oz. meats

Week 1 Friday 2,000 [1,600] (1,200) Calories

Breakfast

Mini Muffins, Yogurt, Juice, Milk
2 orange-cranberry mini muffins [(1)]
6 oz. nonfat, artificially sweetened strawberry yogurt (0)
6 fl. oz. orange juice [(4 fl. oz.)]
8 fl. oz. nonfat milk

Lunch

Turkey, Swiss, and Cranberry Wrap, Side Salad, Peach
turkey, Swiss, and cranberry wrap: 1 whole wheat flour tortilla [(½)],
    spread with ¼ c cranberry sauce (1 T), layered with 3 oz. turkey
    breast [(2 oz.)] and 1 oz. Swiss cheese [(0.6 oz.)]
side salad: 1 c greens and mixed vegetables topped with 1 T oil and
    vinegar dressing
1 medium peach [(small)]

Snack

Cottage Cheese, Walnuts, Plum
4 oz. cottage cheese, 1% fat, no salt added
¼ c walnuts [(1 T)]
1 medium plum [(small)]

Dinner

Pork Chop with Baked Sweet Potato, Applesauce, Asparagus,
    Dinner Salad
5 oz. pork loin chop [(3 oz.)]
1 c baked sweet potato (½)
½ c applesauce, unsweetened
1 c asparagus
dinner salad: 1½ c lettuce and mixed vegetables, topped with 2 T
    French dressing [(1 T)]

DASH servings: 1 whole grain, 4 fruits, 6+ vegetables, 3+ dairy, 1 nuts, 8 oz.
meats

Week 1 Saturday 2,000 [1,600] (1,200) Calories

Breakfast

English Muffin with Cheese, Melon, Juice, Milk

1 cinnamon-raisin English muffin (½), topped with 1 Light
Laughing Cow™ Creamy Spreadable Cheese

6 oz. honeydew melon [(4 oz.)]

6 oz. orange tangerine juice [(4 fl. oz.)]

8 fl. oz. nonfat milk

Lunch

Colorful Beef Tacos, Peach

3 taco shells [(2)], filled with 3 oz. Extra Lean Taco Filling* [(2 oz.)]
and topped with 1 oz. low-sodium, low-fat cheddar cheese [(0.6 oz.)],
diced red tomatoes, shredded romaine lettuce, shredded carrots,
and shredded red cabbage

1 medium peach [(small)]

Snack

Apple, Popcorn, Cheese

1 medium Delicious apple [(small)]

2 c popcorn (0)

1 light string cheese

Dinner

Steak, Baked Potato, Broccoli, Salad

4 oz. broiled T-bone steak [(3 oz.)]

1 baked potato (0)

½ c broccoli

dinner salad: 1½ c greens and mixed vegetables, topped with 2 T
Thousand Island dressing [(1 T)]

1 slice whole wheat bread [(0)], topped with 1 t soft, unsalted
margarine [(0)]

6 oz. nonfat, artificially sweetened peach yogurt

DASH servings: 5 whole grains, 4 fruits, 5 vegetables, 3+ dairy, 1 nuts, 7 oz.
meats

Week 1 Sunday 2,000 [1,600] (1,200) Calories

Breakfast
Southwestern Egg White Omelet, Bagel, Cheese, Juice, Milk
*Southwestern Egg White Omelet**
½ poppy seed bagel, topped with Laughing Cow™ Light Spreadable Cheese
6 oz. fresh squeezed orange juice [(4 fl. oz.)]
8 fl. oz. nonfat milk

Lunch
Grilled Cheese with Tomato, Cucumber Salad, Peaches
grilled cheese: 2 slices whole grain bread (1), 1 oz. low-sodium, low-fat Swiss cheese [(0.6 oz.)], 2 slices tomato
¾ c sliced cucumber topped with 1 T nonfat, no added salt, Italian dressing
1 cup sliced peaches, canned in juice [(½ c)]

Snack
Yogurt, Peanuts, Cantaloupe
6 oz. nonfat, artificially sweetened vanilla yogurt
¼ c peanuts, dry roasted, unsalted [(1 T)]
6 oz. cantaloupe [4 oz.] (0)

Dinner
Roasted Chicken with Potatoes, Vegetables, Pudding, Pear
1 serving *Roasted Chicken with Potatoes, Carrots, and Brussels Sprouts**
½ c chocolate pudding (0)
1 medium pear [(small)]

DASH servings: 2 whole grains, 5 fruits, 5+ vegetables, 3+ dairy, 1 nuts, 8 oz. meats

Week 2

Week 2 Monday 2,000 [1,600] (1,200) Calories

Breakfast

Scrambled Eggs, Toast, Pineapple, Juice, Milk

quick scramblers: in microwave-safe dish, sprayed with nonstick cooking spray, cook ½ c egg substitutes [(¼ c)], 2 minutes on high.

2 slices whole wheat toast [(1)], topped with 4 t orange marmalade [(2 t)]

6 oz. pineapple [(4 oz.)]

6 oz. orange juice [(4 fl. oz.)]

8 fl. oz. nonfat milk

Lunch

Chicken Waldorf salad, with Roll, Italian Coleslaw, Milk, Strawberry Gelatin, Plum

½ c *Chicken Waldorf Salad** [(1/3 c)]

1 whole wheat dinner roll

1 c *Italian coleslaw** [(¼ c)]

8 fl. oz. nonfat milk

½ c artificially sweetened strawberry gelatin

1 medium plum [(small)]

Snack

Banana and Yogurt

1 medium banana [(small)]

6 oz. nonfat, artificially sweetened strawberry-banana yogurt

Dinner

Grilled Tilapia with Potatoes, Asparagus, Salad, Frozen Yogurt

3 oz. grilled tilapia

1 c potatoes (½ c)

1 c asparagus

dinner salad: 1½ c greens and mixed vegetables, topped with 2 T oil and vinegar dressing [(1 T)]

1 c artificially sweetened, nonfat strawberry frozen yogurt (½ c)

DASH servings: 3 whole grains, 4+ fruits, 6 vegetables, 4 dairy, 8 oz. meats

Week 2 Tuesday 2,000 [1,600] (1,200) Calories

Breakfast

English Muffin, Peanut Butter, Yogurt, Orange, Milk

1 mixed grain English muffin [(½)], topped with 1 T natural peanut butter [(2 t)]

6 oz. nonfat, artificially sweetened strawberry banana yogurt

1 medium orange [(small)]

8 fl. oz. nonfat milk

Lunch

Veggie Burger, with Fries, Coleslaw, Banana

veggie burger: whole wheat hamburger bun (0) with grilled vegetable burger patty, soy based, topped with 1oz. low-sodium, low-fat Swiss cheese [(0.6 oz.)], 2 slices red tomato, ¼ c shredded romaine lettuce

1 serving *Oven Potato Fries** (½)

½ c coleslaw

1 medium banana [(small)]

Snack

Cottage Cheese, Pear, Walnuts

4 oz. cottage cheese, no salt added, 1% fat

1 medium pear

¼ c walnuts [(1 T)]

Dinner

Roast Chicken Breast, Baked Potato, Honey Glazed Carrots, Salad, and Frozen Yogurt

4 oz. roasted chicken breast [(3 oz.)]

1 baked potato (½)

1 c honey glazed carrots

dinner salad: 1½ c greens and mixed vegetables, topped with 2 T Italian dressing [(1 T)]

½ c artificially sweetened, nonfat chocolate frozen yogurt (0)

DASH servings: 4 whole grains, 3 fruits, 6+ vegetables, 4 dairy, 1 beans, 1 nuts, 4 oz. meats

Week 2 Wednesday 2,000 [1,600] (1,200) Calories

Breakfast

Oatmeal, Banana, Toast, Grapefruit, Milk

½ c instant oatmeal, unsweetened, topped with 1 medium
   sliced banana [(½)]

1 slice whole wheat toast (0), topped with 2 t strawberry preserves (0)

6 oz. red grapefruit [(4 oz.)]

8 fl. oz. nonfat milk

Lunch

Soup, Cheese & Crackers, Salad, Yogurt, Apple

1 c low-sodium vegetable beef soup (¾ c)

1 oz. low-sodium, low-fat Swiss cheese [(0.6 oz.)], with 6 low-salt whole
   wheat crackers (4)

side salad: 1 c greens and mixed vegetables, topped with 2 T buttermilk
   ranch dressing [(1 T)]

6 oz. nonfat, artificially sweetened peach yogurt

1 medium Gala apple [(small)]

Snack

Cheese, Peach

1 piece light string cheese

1 medium peach [(small)]

Dinner

Pork Chop, Scalloped Potatoes, Green Beans, Carrot-Raisin Salad,
   Walnuts, Milk

4 oz. broiled pork loin chop [(3 oz.)]

½ c scalloped potatoes

1 c green beans

½ c carrot-raisin salad (¼ c), mixed with ¼ c walnuts [(1 T)]

8 fl. oz. nonfat milk

DASH servings: 3 whole grains, 4 fruits, 7 vegetables, 4+ dairy, 1 nuts, 4 oz.
meats

Week 2 Thursday 2,000 [1,600] (1,200) Calories

Breakfast

Cereal, Cantaloupe, Orange Juice, Milk

1½ oz. raisin bran cereal

6 oz. cantaloupe [(4 oz.)]

6 oz. orange juice [(4 fl. oz.)]

8 fl. oz. nonfat milk

Lunch

Grilled Cheese, Salad, Raw Veggies, Pear

grilled cheese with tomato, made with 2 slices whole grain bread, 1 oz. low-sodium, low-fat cheddar cheese, and 2 slices tomato

side salad: 1 c greens and mixed vegetables, topped with 2 T French dressing [1 T] (2 T fat-free dressing)

8 baby carrots

2 celery stalks

1 medium pear [(small)]

Snack

Strawberry Smoothie and Almonds

smoothie: 8 fl. oz. nonfat milk and 6 oz. strawberries [(4 oz.)]

¼ c almonds [(1 T)]

Dinner

Caribbean Chicken, Rice, Cheesy Broccoli, Salad

1 serving *Caribbean Chicken**

1 c long grain white rice

cheesy broccoli: ½ c broccoli, topped with melted 1 oz. low-sodium, low-fat cheddar cheese [(0.6 oz.)]

dinner salad: 1½ c greens and mixed vegetables, topped with 2 T honey mustard dressing [(1 T)]

DASH servings: 3 whole grains, 5 fruits, 5 vegetables, 3 dairy, 1 nuts, 7 oz. meats

Week 2 Friday 2,000 [1,600] (1,200) Calories

Breakfast

Cereal, Banana, Milk, Juice

1 oz. Cheerios™ topped with sliced banana [(½)]

6 fl. oz. orange-strawberry banana juice [(4 fl. oz.)]

8 fl. oz. nonfat milk

Lunch

Tuna Pita, Salad, Grapes

tuna in a pita: ½ whole wheat pita bread (0), ½ c *low-sodium tuna salad* (1/3 c), 2 slices red tomato, handful of radish sprouts

side salad: 1 c greens and mixed vegetables, topped with 2 T blue cheese dressing with Roquefort cheese [(1 T)]

6 oz. grapes [(4 oz.)]

Snack

Peanuts, Plum

¼ c peanuts, dry roasted, unsalted [(1 T)]

1 medium plum [(small)]

Dinner

Cheeseburger, Coleslaw, Veggies, Sundae

extra lean cheeseburger: 4 oz. 95%-lean ground beef [(3 oz)], topped with 1 oz. low-sodium, low-fat Swiss cheese [(0.6 oz.)], 2 slices tomato, and lettuce on a hamburger bun

½ c coleslaw (¼ c)

1 c broccoli, carrots, and cauliflower

sundae: 1 c raspberries [¾ c] (½ c) on 6 oz. nonfat, artificially sweetened vanilla yogurt

DASH servings: 2 whole grains, 4 fruits, 4+ vegetables, 3 dairy, 1 nuts, 7 oz. meats

Week 2 Saturday 2,000 [1,600] (1,200) Calories

Breakfast

Bagel with Cheese, Strawberries, Hot Chocolate, Juice

½ whole grain bagel spread with 1 Light Laughing Cow™
Spreadable Cheese™

6 oz. strawberries [(4 oz.)]

hot chocolate: 8 fl. oz. nonfat milk, 1 heaping teaspoon dry, unsweetened cocoa powder, and 2 packages of Splenda™

6 fl. oz. orange juice [(4 oz.)]

Lunch

Bean and Cheese Burrito, Salad, Pear

1 bean and cheese burrito (½), topped with ¼ oz. shredded low-sodium
Colby cheese, topped with 4 oz. mango salsa

½ cup Mexicali corn

side salad: 1 c lettuce salad with tomatoes and carrots, topped with
1 T pine nuts, and 1 T oil and vinegar dressing

1 medium pear [(small)]

Snack

Latte, Cookies, Fruit Salad

coffee latte, made with 8 fl. oz. nonfat milk and 2 fl. oz. espresso

2 sugar cookies

½ c fruit salad [(0)]

Dinner

New York Strip Steak, Asparagus, Dinner Salad, Peach-Apple Crisp

4 oz. New York strip steak [(3 oz.)]

1 c asparagus

dinner salad: 1½ c greens and mixed vegetables, topped with 2 T oil
and vinegar dressing [(1 T)]

½ c peach-apple crisp, topped with ½ c nonfat, artificially sweetened
vanilla frozen yogurt [¼ c] (0)

DASH servings: 3 whole grains, 5 fruits, 5 vegetables, 5 dairy, 1 beans, 1 nuts,
4 oz. meats

Week 2 Sunday 2,000 [1,600] (1,200) Calories

Breakfast

California Scramble, Pineapple, Juice, Latte

California scramble: 1 whole wheat flour tortilla, filled with ½ c scrambled egg substitutes (¼ c), topped with 3 avocado slices (2), and 2 oz. salsa

6 oz. pineapple [(4 oz.)]

6 fl. oz. orange juice [(4 fl. oz.)]

coffee latte: 2 fl. oz. espresso and 8 fl. oz. nonfat milk

Lunch

Roast Beef and Swiss on Rye, Raw Veggies, Salad, Milk, Peach

roast beef and Swiss on rye: 3 oz. lean roast beef [(2 oz.)], 1 oz. low-sodium, low-fat Swiss cheese [(0.6 oz.)], on 2 slices rye bread [(1)] with mustard

8 baby carrots

6 radishes

side salad: 1 c greens and mixed vegetables, topped with 2 T oil and vinegar dressing [(1 T)]

8 fl. oz. nonfat milk

1 medium peach [(small)]

Snack

Tomato Bisque with Crackers and Tangerine

3/4 c low-sodium tomato bisque soup (½ c) with 6 low-salt crackers (2)

1 medium tangerine [(small)]

Dinner

Pile It On! Chili and Sundae

1 c *Pile It On! Chili** (¾ c), topped with 1 oz. low-sodium, low-fat cheddar cheese [(0.6 oz.)], 2 T fat-free sour cream, and *Baked Corn Tortilla Strips**

sundae: ½ c nonfat, artificially sweetened frozen yogurt, topped with 6 oz. raspberries [(4 oz.)]

DASH servings: 3 whole grains, 6 fruits, 4 vegetables, 3+ dairy, 1 nuts, 7 oz. meats

Week 3

Week 3 Monday 2,000 [1,600] (1,200) Calories

Breakfast

Cereal, Strawberries, Toast, Juice, Milk
1 oz. Special K™, topped with 6 oz. strawberries [(4 oz.)]
1 slice whole wheat toast, topped with 2 t strawberry jam
6 fl. oz. freshly squeezed orange juice [(4 fl. oz.)]
8 fl. oz. nonfat milk

Lunch

Turkey and Swiss on Rye, Carrots, Coleslaw, Orange
turkey and Swiss on rye: 3 oz. roasted turkey breast [(2 oz.)], 1 oz.
  low-sodium, low-fat Swiss cheese [(0.6)] on 2 slices rye bread [(1)]
1 c sliced carrots
1 c coleslaw [½ c] (¼ c)
1 medium navel orange [(small)]

Snack

Gelatin, Cottage Cheese, Nectarine
½ c artificially sweetened strawberry gelatin
4 oz. cottage cheese, no salt added, 1% fat
1 medium nectarine [(small)]

Dinner

Lean, Meaty Spaghetti, Asparagus, Salad, Wine, Frozen Yogurt
1 c *Lean, Meaty Spaghetti Sauce** [(¾ c)] on 1½ c spaghetti [(1 c)]
1 c asparagus
dinner salad: 1½ c greens and mixed vegetables, topped with 2 T oil
  and vinegar dressing [(1 T)]
4 fl. oz. red wine [(0)]
½ c nonfat, artificially sweetened frozen yogurt (0)

DASH servings: 4 whole grains, 4 fruits, 6+ vegetables, 3 dairy, 6 oz. meats

Week 3 Tuesday 2,000 [1,600] (1,200) Calories

Breakfast

Cereal, English Muffin, Honeydew, Juice, Milk

1 oz. Honey Nut Cheerios™

½ raisin-cinnamon English muffin (0), topped with 1 t soft margarine, unsalted (0)

6 oz. honeydew [(4 oz.)]

6 fl. oz. orange juice [(4 fl. oz.)]

8 fl. oz. nonfat milk

Lunch

Tuna and Swiss Sandwich, Salad, Peach

tuna salad and Swiss Sandwich: ½ c *low-sodium tuna salad** [(1/3 c)], 1 oz. low-sodium, low-fat Swiss cheese [(0.6 oz.)], on 2 slices whole wheat bread [(1)]

salad: 1 c greens and mixed vegetables, topped with 2 T Thousand Island dressing [(1 T)]

1 medium peach [(small)]

Snack

Yogurt, Pecans, Strawberries

6 oz. nonfat, artificially sweetened strawberry kiwi yogurt

¼ c pecans, unsalted [(1 T)]

6 oz. strawberries [(4 oz.)]

Dinner

Pasta e Fagioli alla Venezia, Caprese Salad, Pears

*Pasta e Fagioli alla Venezia** (½ serving)

Caprese salad: 1 oz. sliced fresh mozzarella alternated with the slices of 1 tomato, dressed with 1 T extra virgin olive oil and 1 T balsamic vinegar, topped with 1 leaf fresh basil, cut into thin strips

½ c sliced Bartlett pears

DASH servings: 3 whole grains, 5 fruits, 3 vegetables, 4 dairy, 1 nuts, 1 beans, 3 oz. meats

Week 3 Wednesday 2,000 [1,600] (1,200) Calories

Breakfast
Blueberry Muffin, Cheese, Cantaloupe, Juice, Milk
1 small blueberry muffin
1 piece light string cheese
6 oz. cantaloupe [(4 oz.)]
6 oz. orange-tangerine juice [(4 fl. oz.)]
8 fl. oz. nonfat milk

Lunch
Lean Cheeseburger, Coleslaw, Veggies, Apple
cheeseburger: 3 oz. extra lean ground sirloin [(2 oz.)], broiled, topped
    with 1 oz. reduced-fat, reduced-sodium Swiss cheese [(0.6 oz.)], on
    a whole wheat hamburger bun, with 1 T yellow mustard, 1T
    ketchup
½ c coleslaw (¼ c)
½ c broccoli and carrots
1 medium Golden Delicious apple [(small)]

Snack
Raw Pepper Strips Dipped in Guacamole
1 c sliced bell pepper strips, dipped in 4 T guacamole (2 T)

Dinner
Pork Chop, Sweet Potato, Peas, Salad, Yogurt Sundae
*Peach-Mustard Glazed Pork Chop** [(3 oz.)]
1 c baked sweet potato (½ c)
1 c green peas (½ c)
dinner salad: 1½ c greens and mixed vegetables, topped with 2 T oil
    and vinegar dressing [(1 T)]
sundae: 1 c nonfat, artificially sweetened frozen vanilla yogurt [(½ c)],
    topped with 1 c mixed raspberries and blackberries [(½ c)]

DASH servings: 2 whole grains, 4 fruits, 7 vegetables, 4 dairy, 6 oz. meats

Week 3 Thursday 2,000 [1,600] (1,200) Calories

Breakfast

Oatmeal with Applesauce, English Muffin, Yogurt, Juice

½ c oatmeal, mixed with ½ c applesauce [(¼ c)], unsweetened, and sprinkled with cinnamon

½ whole wheat English muffin (0), topped with 1 t raspberry jam (0)

6 oz. nonfat, artificially sweetened vanilla yogurt

6 fl. oz. pineapple juice [(4 fl. oz.)]

Lunch

Chicken Waldorf Salad topped with Walnuts, Roll, Carrots, Milk, Cantaloupe

½ c *Chicken Waldorf Salad** [(1/3 c)] topped with 1 T chopped walnuts

1 small whole wheat dinner roll (0)

8 baby carrots

1 c *Italian coleslaw** [½ c] (¼ c)

8 fl. oz. nonfat milk

6 oz. cantaloupe [(4 oz.)]

Snack

Cheese, Kiwi

1 piece light string cheese

2 kiwifruit [(1)]

Dinner

Roasted Chicken Breast, Baked Potato, Asparagus, Tomato Spinach Salad, Apple Crisp

4 oz. roasted chicken breast [(3 oz.)]

½ medium baked potato

1 c asparagus

tomato spinach salad: 1c baby spinach, 1 tomato, wedged, drizzled with 1 T olive oil and balsamic vinegar

apple crisp (0), topped with ½ c nonfat, artificially sweetened vanilla frozen yogurt (0)

DASH servings: 3 whole grains, 5 fruits, 6 vegetables, 3 dairy, ½ nuts, 7 oz. meats

Week 3 Friday 2,000 [1,600] (1,200) Calories

Breakfast

Chocolate Glazed Doughnut, Banana, Juice, Latte

1 chocolate glazed cake doughnut

1 banana [(½)]

6 fl. oz. orange juice [(4 fl. oz.)]

coffee latte: 2 fl. oz. espresso and 8 fl. oz. nonfat milk

Lunch

Vegetarian Dog, Chips, Cucumber Salad, Veggies, Milk, Watermelon

vegetarian dog: whole wheat hot dog bun, soy-based hot dog, topped
with yellow mustard

1 oz. no salt potato chips [(0)]

½ c cucumber slices, dipped in 2 T ranch dressing [(1 T)]

8 baby carrots

8 grape tomatoes

8 fl. oz. nonfat milk

6 oz. watermelon [(4 oz.)]

Snack

Apple dipped in Peanut Butter

1 medium sliced apple [(small)] dipped in 2 T natural peanut butter
[(1 T)]

Dinner

Veggie-Cheese Pizza, Salad, Trifle

2 slices cheese pizza (1), topped with green peppers, tomato, and
mushrooms

salad: 1½ c greens and mixed vegetables, topped with 2 T nonfat Italian
dressing, no salt added

trifle: ½ c custard, topped with ¼ c sliced strawberries and ½ sliced
banana (¼), and 2 T whipped cream [(0)]

DASH servings: 2 whole grains, 5 fruits, 6 vegetables, 4 dairy, 1 nuts, 1 beans

Week 3 Saturday 2,000 [1,600] (1,200) Calories

Breakfast
Waffles, Maple Syrup, Breakfast Patty, Banana, Orange Juice, Milk
2 low-fat whole wheat waffles, topped with ¼ c reduced calorie maple syrup
1 veggie (soy-based) breakfast patty
1 banana [(½)]
6 fl. oz. orange juice [(4 fl. oz.)]
8 fl. oz. nonfat milk

Lunch
Oriental Chicken Salad on Snow Pea Pods, Milk, Plum
¾ c oriental chicken salad [(½ c)] on a bed of 1 c snow pea pods
8 fl. oz. nonfat milk
1 medium plum [(small)]

Snack
Yogurt, Cashews
6 oz. nonfat, artificially sweetened blueberry yogurt
¼ c cashews, unsalted [(1 T)]

Dinner
Halibut in Balsamic Reduction, on a bed of Smashed Red Potatoes, Brussels Sprouts, Salad, Brownie
3 oz. *Halibut in Balsamic Reduction** on a bed of ½ c *Smashed Red Potatoes** (0)
1 c Brussels sprouts
dinner salad: 1½ c greens and mixed vegetables, topped with 2 T oil and vinegar dressing [(1 T)]
brownie (0)

DASH servings: 2 whole grains, 3 fruits, 5 vegetables, 3 dairy, 1 nuts, 6 oz. meats

Week 3 Sunday 2,000 [1,600] (1,200) Calories

Breakfast

Bagel and cheese, Cereal, Blueberries, Juice, Milk

½ sesame seed bagel (0), topped with 1 Light Laughing Cow Creamy
    Spreadable Cheese™ (0)

1 c Wheaties™

4 oz. blueberries

6 fl. oz. orange juice [(4 fl. oz.)]

8 fl. oz. nonfat milk

Lunch

PB & J on Wheat, Chicken Noodle Soup, Milk, Pineapple

PB & J: 2 slices whole wheat bread (1), 1 T natural peanut butter (2 t),
    1 T grape jelly (2 t)

1 c low-fat chicken noodle soup, no salt added [(¾ c)]

8 fl. oz. nonfat milk

6 oz. pineapple [(4 oz.)]

Snack

Hot Chocolate and Strawberries

hot chocolate: 8 fl. oz. nonfat milk, 1 t unsweetened cocoa powder,
    and 2 packages of Splenda™

6 oz. strawberries [(4 oz.)]

Dinner

BBQ Beef Sandwich, Oven Fries, Sweet Corn, Italian Coleslaw,
    Chocolate Frozen Yogurt

BBQ sandwich: ½ c beef with barbecue sauce on a whole wheat
    hamburger bun [(0)]

1 serving *Oven Potato Fries** [(½)]

½ c sweet corn

1 c *Italian coleslaw** [(½ c)]

½ c unsweetened applesauce

½ c nonfat, artificially sweetened frozen chocolate yogurt (0)

DASH servings: 5 whole grains, 6 fruits, 3+ vegetables, 3+ dairy, 1 nuts, 3 oz.
meats

Week 4

Week 4 Monday 2,000 [1,600] (1,200) Calories

Breakfast

Cereal and Berries, Toast, Juice, Milk

1 oz. bran flakes, topped with 6 oz. mixed blackberries and raspberries [(4 oz.)]

1 slice whole wheat toast, topped with 2 t raspberry preserves

6 fl. oz. orange juice [(4 fl. oz.)]

8 fl. oz. nonfat milk

Lunch

Lean Roast Beef and Swiss on Rye, Coleslaw, Milk, Cantaloupe

lean roast beef and Swiss: 3 oz. lean roast beef [(2 oz.)], 1 oz. low-sodium, low-fat Swiss cheese [(0.6 oz.)] on 2 slices rye bread [(1)]

½ c Italian Coleslaw*

8 fl. oz. nonfat milk

6 oz. cantaloupe [(4 oz.)]

Snack

Orange, Cashews

1 medium California navel orange [(small)]

¼ c cashews [(1 T)]

Dinner

Chicken Cacciatore, Potato Wedges, Peas, Salad, Italian Bread

1 serving *Chicken Cacciatore**

4 oz. potato wedges

½ c baby sweet peas

dinner salad: 1½ c greens and mixed vegetables, topped with 2 T Italian dressing [(1 T)]

1 slice Italian bread (0), topped with 1 t soft unsalted margarine (0)

DASH servings: 4 whole grains, 4 fruits, 4 vegetables, 4 dairy, 1 nuts, 6 oz. meats

Week 4 Tuesday 2,000 [1,600] (1,200) Calories

Breakfast

Blueberry Waffles, Honeydew, Juice, Latte
2 blueberry waffles (1), topped with 2 T light maple syrup (1 T)
6 oz. honeydew [(4 oz.)]
6 fl. oz. grapefruit juice [(4 fl. oz.)]
latte: 8 fl. oz. nonfat milk and 2 fl. oz. espresso

Lunch

Cobb Salad, Roll, Milk, Strawberries
1½ c Cobb salad with dressing, topped with 2 oz. roasted chicken breast
1 whole wheat dinner roll (0)
8 fl. oz. nonfat milk
6 oz. strawberries [(4 oz.)]

Snack

Yogurt and Almonds
6 oz. nonfat, artificially sweetened strawberry-banana yogurt
¼ c almonds, unsalted [(1 T)]

Dinner

Caribbean Chicken on Rice, Green Beans, Salad
*Caribbean Chicken** on 1 c brown rice (½ c)
1 c green beans, frozen or fresh
dinner salad: 1½ c greens and mixed vegetables, topped with 2 T oil
    and vinegar dressing [(1 T)]

DASH servings: 3 whole grains, 4 fruits, 4 vegetables, 4 dairy, 1 nuts, 6 oz.
meats

Week 4 Wednesday 2,000 [1,600] (1,200) Calories

Breakfast

Grab & Go Toasted Pita Melt, Banana, Juice

grab & go toasted pita melt: ½ whole wheat pita bread, stuffed and
toasted with 1 oz. low-sodium, low-fat Swiss cheese [(0.6 oz.)]

1 banana [(½)]

6 fl. oz. no added salt tomato juice [(4 fl. oz.)]

Lunch

Baked Potato topped with Cheesy Broccoli, Salad, Milk, Plum

1 baked potato (½)

cheesy broccoli: 1 oz. low-sodium, low-fat cheddar cheese [(0.6 oz.)]
melted on top of ½ c broccoli

side salad: 1 c green salad and mixed vegetables, with 2 T oil and
vinegar dressing [(1 T)]

8 fl. oz. nonfat milk

1 medium plum [(small)]

Snack

Apple and Peanut Butter

1 medium Granny Smith apple [(small)], sliced and dipped in
2 T peanut butter [(1 T)]

Dinner

Sloppy Joes, Applesauce, Peas and Carrots, Coleslaw, Yogurt Topped
with Berries

½ c *Sloppy Joes** (1/3 c) on a whole wheat hamburger bun [(0)]

½ c applesauce, unsweetened

1 c peas and carrots 1 c Italian coleslaw [(½ c)]

½ c artificially sweetened, nonfat frozen raspberry yogurt, topped
with 1 c mixed berries [(½ c)]

DASH servings: 3 whole grains, 4 fruits, 7 vegetables, 4 dairy, 1 nuts, 3 oz.
meats

Week 4 Thursday 2,000 [1,600] (1,200) Calories

Breakfast

Grits, Berries, Biscuit, Juice, Milk

½ c grits

1 c raspberries [(½ c)]

1 biscuit (0), topped with 2 t raspberry preserves (0)

6 fl. oz. pineapple juice [(4 fl. oz.)]

8 fl. oz. nonfat milk

Lunch

Pile It On! Chili Topped with Cheddar, Salad, Milk, Apple

1 c *Pile It On! Chili** (2/3 c), topped with 1 oz. low-sodium, low-fat shredded cheddar cheese [(0.6 oz.)]

side salad: 1 c greens and mixed vegetables, 8 grape tomatoes, topped with 2 T oil and vinegar dressing [(1 T)]

8 fl. oz. nonfat milk

1 apple

Snack

Yogurt, Peach, Peanuts

6 oz. nonfat, artificially sweetened peach yogurt

1 medium peach [(small)]

¼ c unsalted peanuts [(1 T)]

Dinner

Chicken Stir-Fry on Rice, Egg Roll, and Strawberries

*Chicken Stir-Fry** on ½ c brown rice

1 chicken egg roll [(0)]

6 oz. strawberries [(4 oz.)]

DASH servings: 2 whole grains, 5 fruits, 5 vegetables, 4 dairy, 1 nuts, 1 beans, 6 oz. meats

Week 4 Friday 2,000 [1,600] (1,200) Calories

Breakfast

Cereal, Blueberries, English Muffin, Juice, Milk

1 oz. shredded wheat, topped with 6 oz. blueberries [(4 oz.)]

½ mixed grain English muffin [(0)], topped with 1 t soft, unsalted margarine [(0)]

6 fl. oz. orange juice [(4 fl. oz.)]

8 fl. oz. nonfat milk

Lunch

Waldorf Stuffed Tomato, Corn bread, Snow Pea Pods, Peach

Waldorf stuffed tomato: 1 c *Tuna Waldorf Salad** [(¾ c)] in a tomato

½ c snow pea pods

1 c side salad with 2 T nonfat, no added salt, Italian dressing

1 slice corn bread (0)

1 medium peach [(small)]

Afternoon snack

Gelatin, Cheese, Apple

½ c artificially sweetened mixed fruit gelatin

1 oz. Light Baby Bel™ cheese

1 medium Gala apple [(small)]

Dinner

Lean Swiss Cheeseburger, Oven Potato Fries, Broccoli, Coleslaw, Banana Split

Swiss cheeseburger: whole-wheat hamburger bun [(0)], 3 oz. broiled extra lean ground sirloin with 1 oz. low-fat Swiss cheese [(0.6 oz.)]

1 serving *Oven Potato Fries** [(½)]

½ c broccoli

1 c coleslaw [(½ c)]

banana split: ½ c each nonfat, artificially sweetened chocolate and vanilla frozen yogurt (¼ c each), banana (½), 2 T chocolate syrup (1 T)

DASH servings: 4 whole grains, 5 fruits, 6 vegetables, 5 dairy, ½ nuts, 6 oz. meats

Week 4 Saturday 2,000 [1,600] (1,200) Calories

Breakfast
Glazed Doughnut, Banana, Orange Juice, Latte
1 glazed doughnut
1 banana [(½)]
6 fl. oz. freshly squeezed orange juice [(4 fl. oz.)]
latte: 2 fl. oz. espresso and 8 fl. oz. nonfat milk

Lunch
Soup and Half Sandwich, Coleslaw, Milk, Cantaloupe
half sandwich: 1 slice whole-wheat bread, ½ c chicken salad [(1/3 c)]
¾ c low-sodium split pea soup
1 c *Italian Coleslaw** [(½ c)]
8 fl. oz. nonfat milk
6 oz. cantaloupe [(4 oz.)]
1 c strawberries [(½ c)]

Snack
Yogurt, Popcorn, Apple
6 oz. nonfat, artificially sweetened blueberry yogurt
2 c light microwave popcorn (0)
1 medium McIntosh apple [(small)]

Dinner
Grilled Shrimp, Mixed Vegetables, Salad, Milk, Peach-Topped Frozen
    Yogurt
4 oz. grilled shrimp kebobs [(3 oz.)], with ½ c pepper chunks
1 c mixed cauliflower, broccoli, and carrots
dinner salad: 1½ c greens and mixed vegetables, topped with 2 T oil and
    vinegar dressing [(1 T)]
8 fl. oz. nonfat milk
½ c artificially sweetened, nonfat vanilla frozen yogurt, topped with 1
    medium peach, sliced [(small)]

DASH servings: 3 whole grains, 5 fruits, 5 vegetables, 4 dairy, 1 nuts, and 7 oz.
meats

Week 4 Sunday 2,000 [1,600] (1,200) Calories

Breakfast

Scrambled Eggs and Bacon, Toast, Hot Chocolate, Raspberries, Juice

2 scrambled eggs [(1)]

2 slices bacon [(0)]

2 slices whole-wheat toast [1] (0), topped with 4 t raspberry jam [2 t] (0)

hot chocolate: 8 fl. oz. nonfat milk, 1 t cocoa powder, and 2 packages Splenda™

1 c raspberries [(½ c)]

6 fl. oz. freshly squeezed orange juice [(4 fl. oz.)]

Lunch

Chicken Quesadilla, Salad, Cantaloupe

chicken quesadilla: 1 whole-wheat tortilla [(½)], topped with 3 oz. roasted chicken breast [(2 oz.)], and 1 oz. low-sodium, low-fat Colby Jack cheese [(0.6 oz.)]. Fold tortilla over and heat in toaster oven, until cheese is melted. Top with 2 T guacamole [(1 T)].

side salad: 1 c green salad with mixed vegetables, 2 T oil and vinegar dressing [(1 T)]

6 oz. cantaloupe [(4 oz.)]

Snack

Banana Strawberry Smoothie

smoothie: 8 fl. oz. nonfat milk, banana [(½)], 1 c strawberries [(4 oz.)]

Dinner

Meat Loaf, Mashed Potatoes, Broccoli, Salad, Frozen Yogurt

3 oz. meat loaf

½ c home-style mashed potatoes

½ c broccoli

dinner salad: 1½ c greens, 2 T oil and vinegar dressing [(1 T)]

½ c artificially sweetened, nonfat chocolate frozen yogurt

DASH servings: 3 whole grains, 5 fruits, 4 vegetables, 3+ dairy, 9 oz. meats

CHAPTER 4

MENU GUIDE—DASH MEALS AWAY FROM HOME

Staying on track with any healthy eating plan can be a challenge when you are away from home. With a little advance planning, however, you can still hit the mark with the DASH diet without being overly stressed.

If you are lucky, you eat many of your meals-away-from-home at real (sit-down) restaurants. Many of us rely on take-out or fast food restaurants too often, but we can still find foods that fit into the DASH Diet Action Plan. Travel presents special concerns, but this is a part of real life, so we need to have DASH tips for trips too. And special events can trip you up, if you don't think, and plan beforehand.

Restaurant Meals

At restaurants, there are three key rules to help you stay on track with portion size. Share. Divide and conquer. Bag it. These tips, and a few more, will help you stay the course.

1. **Split up**. If you have an agreeable spouse, partner, or friend, split entrées, large salads, and desserts.

2. **Bon appetizer**. Choose an item from the appetizer section of the menu instead of a main course.

3. **Basta pasta**. Basta is Italian for Enough! However, most Italian restaurants serve more than enough, especially, pasta. It makes it look like you are getting good value, but you aren't getting lots of the really good stuff. To increase the DASH quotient, ask to have the sauce on steamed vegetables instead of pasta. Save the grain servings for the bread, if it is really good. If you do have pasta, ask them to serve only a small portion, and then save the remainder to take home for several more meals.

4. **Bag it**. If you really can't stop eating the food that is in front of you, ask the server to bag half (or more) before he or she brings it out. One of my clients found she could successfully cut her calories by putting half of her meal on a bread plate. As long as it wasn't on her plate, she could avoid overeating. Then she would ask to have the leftover portion wrapped to take home for another meal.

5. **Avoid portion distortion**. Choose your portion size. Many short women who want to lose weight find that half-sized portions are still too big to fit into their calorie allotment. You may find that one-third or a quarter of a serving is more appropriate. Decide, before you start to eat.

6. **Just desserts**. Order just one dessert for four people. This makes it easy to avoid overdoing.

7. **Side order of veggies**. Fill up on non-starchy vegetables

to maximize the DASH potential of your diet, and support losing weight. Order extra vegetables.

8. **Prime isn't best.** When you are trying to follow a moderate fat diet, lower your cholesterol, or lose weight, prime meats don't fill the bill. Prime meats have more hidden fat, also referred to as marbling. If you are at a restaurant with only prime meats, choose fish or tenderloin. Tenderloin is a relatively lean cut, often called filet mignon on menus. Choose the petite filet (eight ounces), which will give you a six-ounce portion to eat. If you have already had one serving of meat, fish, or poultry that day, only eat half of what is served at dinner. Save the rest for a meal later in the week. Half of a six-ounce cooked serving is three ounces—a perfect size for the DASH diet.

9. **Bread, bread, everywhere.** If bread is your downfall, tell yourself you will only have whole grain. This will cut down on your bread intake right away. If you do have bread, don't put butter on it! If bread is your weakness and you won't give it up at restaurants, ask the waiter to delay bringing the bread until your salad is served. This will eliminate the mindless bread eating that is typical of many of us at restaurants, while we are waiting for our food to be served.

Fast Food Meals

Fast food makes it a little harder to keep to the DASH diet, but occasional fast food meals can fit into a flexible plan. Most fast food restaurants have salads. Add some grilled chicken, watch your salad dressing portion size, and you have a DASH-friendly meal. If you keep some portable fruit with you, such as apples, tangerines (especially Clementine tangerines in the winter), plums, nectarines, or grapes, you will be able to add fiber and sweetness. Add a carton of skim milk and you will have added several of the key DASH foods to your day, even with fast food meals.

Travel Days

While you are on the road, it may seem difficult to stay with the DASH plan. You may not be able to make every meal DASH-friendly, but you can identify meals where you can be sure to get many of the key DASH foods, and load up when you can. Breakfast is a sure bet for fruit servings and dairy. Even McDonald's has skim milk and orange juice. Many Starbucks and other coffeehouse restaurants (and now even several fast food chains) have fruit cups in addition to juice. Add a skim latte or a skim hot chocolate, and you have a nonfat dairy serving.

At sit-down restaurants, order an omelet made with egg whites or egg substitutes, and include peppers, onions, and mushrooms. Many restaurants now offer fresh fruit instead of toast or potatoes for low-carb diners at breakfast. This is a great way to keep your calories under control while you are on the road. At lunch grab a salad and grilled chicken if you are fast fooding it. If you get to eat at a real restaurant, you can have a side salad and extra vegetables.

For snacks, stop at a grocery store and get some low-fat portable cheese, a small bag of nuts, and some fruit. In the evening, look for restaurants where you can order vegetable side dishes, great salads, and foods that are not overly fatty. Many chain restaurants have lighter options, and most local restaurants will have vegetable sides. Restaurants that cater to low-carb diners will be happy to serve extra vegetables, and may even have fresh fruit for dinner. When you go to the market to buy snacks, buy some extra fruit for your evening dessert.

Special Events

Weddings, christenings, birthday parties, confirmations, bar/bat mitzvahs, and anniversaries are all occasions that bring special challenges in staying with any healthy eating plan. The best strategy is to choose a few special items as indulgences at the party, and try to keep the rest of the day relatively on target with your DASH plan.

Restaurants

Some of the information here may feel repetitive, however many people jump around in books, looking for specific information. My apologies in advance if you feel that you have already seen some of the advice provided here.

Starbucks and Other Coffeehouses

Choose a latte made with eight ounces of skim milk. This gives you a full serving of milk. If you don't drink coffee, order hot chocolate made with skim milk, without whipped cream. Most Starbucks locations have fruit cups. If you want a pastry, choose a bagel, but only eat half. Most bagels equal four to five servings of grains. If you do choose a bagel, a cinnamon-raisin bagel provides plenty of flavor and has creaminess without needing the extra calories and saturated fat of cream cheese.

Watch out for large juice containers that hold two to two-and-a-half servings of fruit (DASH serving sizes are six ounces, regardless of the serving size on the label). I generally recommend that people limit themselves to one serving of juice each day. Juice is less filling than fruit, making it easy to overdo calories. Juice also does not contain the beneficial fiber of fruit, and ounce for ounce, has more sugar than regular pop.

Italian

The best choices on an Italian menu are the vegetables. There are so many wonderful choices that will boost the DASH-quotient of your meal. A variety of salads and many pasta toppings provide you with the opportunity to choose from many different plant-based foods. The chicken and seafood dishes give you many choices for lean protein. Olive oil-based dressings provide heart-healthy monounsaturated fats.

Key pitfalls include cream based sauces and full fat cheeses that are high in saturated fats, large pasta serving sizes, and bread. Many restaurants provide four to eight servings of pasta on each plate. If you have eaten two or three pieces of bread before the meal, you can easily consume double the servings of grains you need for that day.

Sometimes I recommend that people ask to have the pasta sauce put on top of vegetables instead of pasta. If you have trouble limiting bread before the meal, ask the server to hold off on the bread until your salad arrives. Bread often triggers mindless eating, and it doesn't fill you up enough to limit intake during the meal. Topping bread with butter or soaking it in olive oil only adds to the calorie overload. Refined bread and pasta don't add any DASH-benefit to the meal, so choosing to limit them does not compromise the diet, and can improve it if you choose more vegetables instead.

If you are having pizza, choose vegetable toppings, and limit yourself to a few slices of thin crust or one slice of thick crust pizza. Start your meal with a good-sized salad to fill you up, and help you avoid overdoing pizza. In Italy, a typical dessert in restaurants is fresh fruit, rather than cannoli or tiramisu. Since only 29% of Americans get even two servings of fruit each day, following the Italian example can be a great idea and provides a satisfying end to a wonderful meal.

Chinese

Just like Italian cuisine, Chinese menus can be rich sources of vegetables. However, they can also be full of hidden fats and loads of extra carbs. To get the maximum DASH benefit, order an extra serving of steamed vegetables. Put some of your entrée on the vegetables rather than on rice. One cup of cooked rice has 200 calories. Many of us have two to three cups of rice at a Chinese restaurant, which can easily put us over our allotment of grain servings and over our calorie limit. And many of the appetizers are loaded with calories. Egg rolls can have as much as 400 to 600 calories *each*! Crab rangoon is loaded with cream cheese; fried pot stickers are equally high in fat (and calories). Choose appetizers that have not been fried to minimize your calorie intake. Steamed appetizers or soup would be a better choice.

American Casual

Many chain restaurants are competing based on providing more value for the money. This usually takes the form of large portions. The first DASH trick is to cut down the portion size. Share with a friend or ask the server to wrap half the meal before he or she brings it out. Then decide if it is still too large. Identify how much you want to eat from the very start, and get it off your plate. Use your bread plate to hold the part that you don't want to eat (at that meal). If it stays on your plate, you will probably eat it. If you like hearty portions, order extra vegetables (without butter, cheese, or too much oil) and fill up on non-starchy vegetables.

Watch out for sautéed or grilled vegetables. They are typically oil-laden and bursting with extra calories. (Grilled vegetables tend to soak up cooking oil like a sponge, unlike grilled meats, which tend to lose fat in the cooking process.)

Restaurant food often has extra-rich flavors due to added toppings, especially those with large amounts of cheese. While cheese is a great calcium-rich DASH food, large amounts of full-fat cheese pile on extra calories and loads of saturated fats. These cheeses can come in salads, on pizza (sometimes stuffed in the crust), in pasta toppings, sandwiches, and on top of meat or

65

chicken. Leave the cheese off the salad and limit portion sizes of the other cheese-rich foods.

Fast Food

The fast food industry has been under attack for causing obesity in children and adults. However, fast food has become a mainstay of American culture in our overscheduled lives. Making smart choices at fast food restaurants can be challenging, but it can be done.

Most restaurants have salads. Choose grilled chicken instead of crispy, and limit the serving size of dressing if you choose a full-fat dressing. If you want a sandwich, choose the smallest burger or a grilled chicken sandwich. If you need to limit grains at this meal, remove half the bun. If the restaurant has a sandwich with lettuce and tomatoes this can be a good choice, but they may be available only on larger sandwiches that have more calories. If you absolutely have to add fries to your meal, order the small serving and throw out half before you start eating (or split it with a friend or your kids). Potatoes are rich in potassium, but you don't need the extra calories from the fat. Some chicken sandwiches have more calories and fat than others, so check the on-line nutrient listings via our links at http://dashdiet.org/health_links.asp. Add a carton of skim milk to increase the DASH benefits of your meal. Some franchises are now offering fresh fruits, so take advantage if they are available.

Since portion size is so critical, you really want to avoid the impulse to "super size" or "biggie size" your meals. At fast food restaurants, we are unlikely to save part of the meal for another day and we tend to eat everything that we purchase. So, reframe your idea of what makes for good value in a meal. Traditionally we consider a meal to be a good value if we get a lot for our money. However, for many of us, this means that we overeat and get fatter from foods that add little nutritional value. A better concept for the DASH diet is to consider good value to be a meal that is rich in fruits, vegetables, low-fat dairy, and lean meats, fish, or poultry. A good-value DASH meal is not heavy in fats or refined carbohydrates. Your first priority is to choose foods that improve your health, not foods that expand your waistline.

Sandwich restaurants seem like a good choice, since the foods are not fried (except for the chips often purchased with the meals). However, they are often unbalanced in terms of the ratio of refined grains to protein. For example a six-inch turkey sub from Subway™ contains three servings of bread and one ounce (one-third of a serving) of turkey. Yes, you can add vegetables, which is great, but you are getting lots of carbs and too little protein. This is a meal that may leave you hungry an hour or two later. A better choice is to order the roasted chicken, which comes in a two-ounce serving size or order double meat, and lose the top part of the bread. Surprisingly, there is no fiber advantage if you compare their "whole wheat" versus the other breads. The key to keeping calories under control in sandwich shops is to watch out for the bread serving size. You also want to avoid eating an entire large bag of chips. These are often the Big Grab™ size, which hold 2½ ounces. Even if you choose baked chips, you are getting lots of calories. Try to limit yourself to a small handful, and toss the rest. Remember, it is more wasteful to consume extra calories and increase your health risk, than to throw away extra food.

Sauces, dressings, and toppings are another source of extra calories. Mustard, ketchup, veggies, salsa, and low-fat mayonnaise are good choices. Since ketchup is high in salt and sugar, you want to limit it to one package rather than pouring it over the entire meal or using it as a dip. Limit use of regular mayonnaise, oil, sour cream, and large servings of regular salad dressing. For example, at salad bars, many people use half a cup or more of salad dressing. Regular dressing has a whopping 500 calories per half-cup. You can avoid overdoing, by avoiding thick dressings, such as Thousand Island. A better choice would be "slippery" dressings, such as Italian, which give good salad coverage with a small amount of dressing—and the excess drips onto the plate. The mayonnaise that tops many sandwiches is three-fourths of an ounce, which adds 160 calories to the sandwich. Request no mayonnaise, or ask them to use only a little. A baked potato topped with broccoli and cheese has fifty-five percent more calories than a plain baked potato. Since a half-cup of broccoli only has twenty-five calories, clearly the extra calories come from the full-fat cheese. Toppings can take a meal that has relatively moderate calories and push it over the top, so limit high-fat extras.

On the Job

Many workplaces make it difficult to stick with a healthy eating plan. Too little time and limited choices make conditions that can lead to overweight and hypertension. However, you can choose to take charge of your health and eat healthy meals, even at work.

Some companies have cafeterias that provide a great way to get more variety. Most cafeterias have some kind of salad bar. Choose mayonnaise-free veggies and fruits. Get a serving of cooked vegetables. Add skim milk or light yogurt. If your cafeteria is lacking in some of your favorites, talk to the manager and make some recommendations. The key DASH foods are healthy choices, and are great for people who are watching their weight. With so many people trying to lose weight or eat more healthfully, you won't be the only one who will appreciate the new choices.

If you have access to a refrigerator at work, stock it with yogurt, fruits, raw veggies, light cheeses, and milk chugs. Or bring a few of these each day in an insulated bag.

Business meetings and coworkers with treats can present challenging obstacles to your DASH plan, especially if you are trying to lose weight. If you bring healthy snacks to work and have regular meals and snacks, you won't be as hungry and will be less likely to be tempted by office treats or birthday cakes.

Hunger leads to diminished resolve when it comes to avoiding empty calorie treats. In the morning, have some light yogurt or fresh fruit before you reach the office, and you won't be tempted to eat several doughnuts or a bagel slathered with cream cheese. Ask meeting planners to include fresh fruits or raw veggies for snacks. Or, you could be the one to bring in a fruit tray or a bowl of apples rather than a box of doughnuts.

If your boss rewards the staff with a pizza party at lunch, try to stick with just one slice, have a piece of fruit, and then eat a smaller dinner with an emphasis on low-calorie veggies. If you see a candy jar that seems to be calling to you, get back to your desk and enjoy a piece of light cheese and fruit, or yogurt and nuts. If your choice is between having nothing versus indulging in diet-busting foods, chances are that you will give in to temptation. Keep healthy snack foods on hand.

The key to watching your weight and following the DASH guidelines is to plan ahead. Think about what you need for the whole day. How will your meals away from home fit into your DASH plan? Restaurant meals are not a surprise, they are typical for most of us. When you know you will be eating out, plan ahead and think about your choices. Do you need some vegetables and low-fat dairy at this meal? Envision what you will order before you look at the menu or stand in line at a fast food place. Then you will be less likely to choose a tempting, but empty calorie meal and you will meet your DASH objectives every day.

DASHboard

Surviving restaurant meals:

1. Plan what you will choose before you go.
2. Manage portion sizes by sharing, choosing smaller servings, or taking half (or more) home. Many entrées and desserts can easily serve three to four people.
3. Choose lean meats, poultry, or fish.
4. Limit bread to whole grains or hold off on the bread basket until your salad arrives.
5. Choose salads at fast-food outlets, and skim milk as a side. Carry portable fruit to round out the meal.
6. On the road, buy fruits; low-fat, individually packaged cheese; and unsalted nuts to complement restaurant meals.

Tracking my Personal DASH Diet Action Plan

Three specific changes I will make at restaurants and/or at work:

_____

_____

_____

_____

_____

CHAPTER 5

DASH YOUR WAY TO WEIGHT LOSS

The DASH diet makes it easy to lose weight. A healthy diet, based on fruits, vegetables, and other key DASH foods, will help you have satisfying meals, without overeating. And, new research shows that including calcium-rich dairy foods in your diet can have special benefits for weight loss. DASH provides the perfect foundation for a weight loss plan.

Losing weight is recommended as one of the key lifestyle changes to help manage high blood pressure. Even greater advantages can be expected when weight loss is combined with the DASH diet. In this chapter, you will learn how to identify your healthy weight, calculate the calories you need to reach that goal, and learn specific weight loss strategies.

Research has shown that foods in the DASH diet can support weight loss. With a diet rich in fruits and vegetables, you can fill up without overdoing calories. Lean meat, fish, and poultry provide satiating protein with fewer calories than higher fat meats. For example, eight ounces of boiled shrimp have the same calories as three ounces of corned beef, while providing more satisfaction. Low-fat dairy foods have significantly lower calories than the higher fat versions they replace. And research suggests that diets rich in dairy calcium promote weight loss, especially helping to reduce the extra fat around your waist.

Being overweight is a primary risk factor for developing high blood pressure. For children and teens, extra weight is even riskier. Parents with high blood pressure who adopt the DASH diet, help their kids significantly by providing the right foods and avoiding calorie-laden meals. Children learn eating patterns by observing their parents. As a parent, you can model healthy behavior, and help your children avoid a lifetime regimen of blood pressure medication. Knowing that your actions are important for the whole family can provide strong motivation to follow through on your own diet and lifestyle changes.

What is a Healthy Weight?

There are many ways to evaluate whether you are at a healthy weight. The Metropolitan Life Weight Tables were used for many years to identify healthy weights. Recently, BMI (body mass index, which shows the relation of weight to height) has become an important tool for assessing healthy weight. Body fat percentage is another indicator of fitness (or fatness). And some health professionals believe that a healthy weight is the weight at which you do not have health issues, or at least none related to your weight.

In 1998, the National Institutes of Health issued new guidelines for healthy weight, based on BMI. The guidelines were developed to provide information on the ratio of weight to height, associated with lower risk of disease. BMI is based on a formula of weight in kilograms divided by height in meters, squared. The table on page 76 lets you find your BMI (without a calculator) and shows you where your weight falls in terms of health risks. It is important to realize that not everyone who is in the elevated risk category is truly at higher risk for disease. The BMI tables reflect generalized risk for large numbers of people, but not for each individual. For example, a sedentary person who is at a healthy weight might have a higher risk for disease than someone who is overweight but physically fit. And, a football player might appear to be overweight by the BMI tables, although he is probably not "over fat."

A BMI of less than 19 is considered to be underweight, 19 - 25 is a healthy weight, 26 - 30 is overweight, 31 - 39 is obese, and a BMI greater than 40 is considered to be very obese.

Fitness (or fatness) can be measured by looking at body fat percentage, which can be evaluated in several ways. In a research setting (and in some physician offices), body fat can be measured by DEXA (dual emission X-ray analysis), which can be done on the same equipment that is used for performing bone mineral density scans. This is considered to be the most reliable procedure. Inexpensive bio-electrical impedance analysis (BIA) devices for home use can provide useful information and are built-in to some home scales or are available in a handheld device that is gripped like a steering wheel. Underwater weighing is another way to measure body fat and is performed at some health clubs. Healthy body fat percentages are shown in the following table. The average American man has 24.5% body fat, and the average woman has 33%.

Waist size is another healthy weight indicator. Waist circumference is used to evaluate whether you might be at increased risk for certain diseases. You may be familiar with the concept of apple versus pear physiques. People who carry most of their

BMI (Body Mass Index)

Find your height in inches at left, follow across to your weight, and then look to the top of the column to find your BMI.

Height (inches)	18	19	20	21	22	23	24	25	26	27	28	29	30	31	32	33	34	35	36	37	38	39	40
58	86	91	96	100	105	110	115	120	124	129	134	139	144	148	153	158	163	167	172	177	182	187	191
59	89	94	99	104	109	114	119	124	129	134	139	144	149	153	158	163	168	173	178	183	188	193	198
60	92	97	102	108	113	118	123	128	133	138	143	148	154	159	164	169	174	179	184	189	195	200	205
61	95	101	106	111	116	122	127	132	138	143	148	153	159	164	169	175	180	185	191	196	201	206	212
62	98	104	109	115	120	126	131	137	142	148	153	158	164	169	175	180	186	191	197	202	208	213	219
63	102	107	113	119	124	130	135	141	147	152	158	163	169	175	180	186	192	198	203	209	215	220	226
64	105	111	117	122	128	134	140	146	151	157	163	168	174	181	186	192	198	204	210	216	221	227	233
65	108	114	120	126	132	138	144	150	156	162	168	174	180	186	192	198	204	210	216	222	228	234	240
66	112	118	124	130	136	142	149	155	161	167	173	180	186	192	198	204	211	216	223	229	235	242	248
67	115	121	128	134	140	147	153	160	166	172	179	185	192	198	204	211	217	223	230	236	243	249	255
68	118	125	132	138	145	151	158	164	171	178	184	191	197	204	210	217	224	230	237	243	250	256	263
69	122	129	135	142	149	156	163	169	176	183	190	196	203	210	217	223	230	237	244	251	257	264	271
70	125	132	139	146	153	160	167	174	181	188	195	202	209	216	223	230	237	244	251	258	265	272	279
71	129	136	143	151	158	165	172	179	186	194	201	208	215	222	229	237	244	251	258	265	272	280	287
72	133	140	147	155	162	170	177	184	192	199	206	214	221	229	236	243	251	258	265	273	280	288	295
73	136	144	152	159	167	174	182	189	197	205	212	220	227	235	243	250	258	265	273	280	288	296	303
74	140	148	156	164	171	179	187	195	203	210	218	226	234	241	249	257	265	272	280	288	296	304	312
75	144	152	160	168	176	184	192	200	208	216	224	232	240	248	256	264	272	280	288	296	304	312	320
76	148	156	164	173	181	189	197	205	214	222	230	238	246	255	263	271	279	288	296	304	312	320	329
77	152	160	169	177	186	194	202	211	219	228	236	245	253	261	270	278	287	295	304	312	320	329	337
78	156	164	173	182	190	199	208	216	225	234	242	251	260	268	277	286	294	303	312	320	329	337	346
79	160	169	178	186	195	204	213	222	231	240	249	257	266	275	284	293	302	311	320	328	337	346	355
80	164	173	182	191	200	209	218	228	237	246	255	264	273	282	291	300	309	319	328	337	346	355	364
81	168	177	187	196	205	215	224	233	243	252	261	271	280	289	299	308	317	327	336	345	355	364	373
82	172	182	191	201	210	220	230	239	249	258	268	277	287	296	306	316	325	335	344	354	363	373	383

BMI under 19 Underweight

BMI 19 - 25 Healthy weight

BMI 26-30 Overweight

BMI 31 - 39 Obesity

BMI 40 and above Extreme obesity

Suggested Percent Body Fat Standards for Adults

	Men	Women
Lean	<8	<15
Optimal health	8-15	15-22
Slightly overweight	16-20	23-26
Fat	21-24	27-32
Obese or over fat	25+	32+

extra fat around their waist (apple-shaped) are at higher risk for heart disease, type 2 diabetes, and certain types of cancer, compared to people who carry extra weight in their hips (pear-shaped). If waist circumference is greater than thirty-five inches for women or forty inches for men, it is probably a good idea to lose weight and increase physical activity.

Another concept of healthy weight holds that it is possible to be healthy and yet be heavier than the desirable weight. If you have high blood pressure and you are overweight, then this would not apply to you. You will most likely benefit from some weight reduction. As with most things, we need to use our judgment when deciding on a healthy weight for any specific person.

Deciding on Your Healthy Weight Goal

You can decide what your target weight will be. It will probably be somewhere in the healthy BMI zone. If you have a long way to go, you might set a short-term goal to lose about 10% of your total weight. Many research studies have shown that people can significantly improve their health if they lose 7 to 10% of their body weight.

Your starting weight   _____

Starting date   _____

Your target weight   _____

Date expected to reach   _____

Now that you have selected a target weight, you need to decide how much you can safely lose each week. Typically, nutrition professionals think that women can lose about one or two pounds per week and men can lose two to four pounds per week (perhaps more at the beginning, for people who have a lot to lose). Your goal is to lose fat and maintain muscle. If you lose weight too fast, you may lose muscle and slow down your metabolism. The DASH diet plan, which has plenty of low-fat protein foods, calcium-rich dairy, high fiber fruits, vegetables, and whole grains, will support healthy weight loss.

What Are Your Calorie Needs?

To lose one pound per week, you will need to reduce your calorie intake by 500 calories per day (if you make no activity changes). In order to make your diet plan, you need to estimate your daily calorie needs. There are many sophisticated formulas that can estimate your calorie needs, and even machines to directly evaluate your metabolic rate. For most people, it is practical to estimate needs based on the following guidelines.

Estimating calorie needs for weight maintenance

Activity level	Calories per pound body weight	Calories per kilogram body weight
Sedentary	13.5	30
Moderate	16	35
Heavy	18	40

Multiply your weight by the calories per pound (or kilo-gram), and you will have the amount of daily calories you need to maintain your weight. Then subtract 500 calories in order to lose one pound per week (or 1000 if you want to lose two pounds per week).

Current weight		_____
Calories per pound	X	_____
Calories to maintain	=	_____
Minus calories to lose	-	_____
Target calories	=	_____

Adding exercise to your weight loss program will help you have a more generous calorie allotment, and it will also help lower your blood pressure and improve cardiovascular fitness. See Chapter 6 for more information on the payoff from exercise and specific recommendations to help you meet your goals.

Your target calories will be used to determine the number of servings you need from each of the food groups in the DASH diet. You should not go lower than 1,200 calories per day. Below this intake, it will be difficult to get enough of the key DASH foods, and the diet will probably not provide a healthy balance of foods. Your objective is to improve your health and to have a plan that is sustainable for the long run. Moderate weight loss through healthy eating and exercise will reduce your blood pressure and reduce other health risks, such as cancer and heart disease.

Weight Loss Strategies

There are several important strategies that will help you lose weight. One is to be sure that you are not overeating. This seems obvious, but portion sizes are increasing at restaurants, in convenience foods, packaged foods, and even recipes.

The next section will key you in on how to avoid "portion distortion." Extra calories can also sneak in through foods that are fattening. This also seems obvious, but there are many foods that are "calorie-dense," which means that extra calories are packed into a normal-sized serving.

For example, one national steak house chain provides croissants with their dinner salad. The croissants have 400 or more calories each, compared with 80 calories for a slice of bread. Then the salad is topped with more than an ounce of full-fat cheese and a generous serving of bacon. The salad course alone will contribute at least 1,000 calories to the meal. This example makes it easy to see how Americans are getting fatter without feeling like they are doing anything different.

When you are eating at home, food labels will help you get a handle on how much you eat. Many of the foods that everyone thinks are quite healthful may provide relatively empty calories, without being filling, and can lead to eating more calories than you realize. Chapter 11 provides information to help you decipher the Nutrition Facts on food labels.

Avoid Portion Distortion

Buy a digital scale. No, not for you, for the food! Getting a handle on portion size is the first step in weight loss. If you measure and weigh your foods at home, you will be better able to estimate portion sizes in restaurants.

At home many of us underestimate how much we eat in several ways. Cereal provides a good example, since it is very easy to underestimate portion size. Many cereal bowls hold two or more cups of cereal. And many cereals are quite calorie-dense. It is especially important to read the labels on cereal boxes. A DASH-sized serving is one ounce by weight. Some of the high fiber cereals are the worst in terms of packing a lot of calories in a small serving size. For example, Grape Nuts™ provide 105 calories in a one-ounce serving, which measures only a quarter-cup. A full cup of Grape Nuts™ would provide 420 calories. Bran Buds™ have 70 calories for a one-ounce serving, measuring one-third cup. If you eat one cup for breakfast, you are consuming 210 calories, without the milk. If you prefer more volume, you might want to choose flaked or puffed cereals, such as Grape Nut Flakes™ where a one-ounce serving is seven-eighths of a cup, for 105 calories.

Oatmeal is another source of "portion distortion." A DASH-serving of cooked oatmeal is a half-cup. Pre-packaged instant oatmeal may contain two servings of oatmeal. You can increase the volume of smaller-sized cereal servings by topping them with berries or other sliced fruit. This improves the DASH score of your breakfast, and allows you to sweeten without adding sugar and extra calories.

When you are measuring foods, remember that the serving sizes refer to cooked portions for foods that are normally served cooked. The following table will show you the DASH serving sizes. These are not always the same as the serving sizes on food labels or the diabetic exchanges. A more detailed list is found on our Website at http://dashdiet.org/servingsizes.asp.

Another source of serving size error is confusing weight measures with volume measures. In this book we will call weight measures ounces, and volume measures are called fluid ounces. For example one ounce (by weight) of cereal might be a quarter-cup (two fluid ounces) or one cup (eight fluid ounces). When you weigh the foods with a digital scale, you avoid confusion.

DASH Diet Serving Sizes

Grains, starches	1 slice of bread ½ English muffin or bun ¼ bagel 1 ounce dry cereal ½ cup cooked cereal, pasta, corn, rice
Fruits	6 ounces by weight 6 fluid ounces of juice 1 medium piece of fruit ½ cup canned, frozen fruit ¼ cup dried fruit
Vegetables	½ cup cooked or raw vegetables 1 cup leafy raw vegetables 6 fluid ounces vegetable juice
Dairy	8 fluid ounces (1 cup) milk, yogurt 1½ ounces of cheese ½ cup cottage cheese
Meats, fish, poultry	2½-3½ ounces, cooked
Eggs	1 egg 2 egg whites 1 fluid ounce egg-substitute
Beans	¼ cup cooked beans, lentils, or peas
Nuts	¼ cup or 1 ounce nuts 2 Tbsp or 1 ounce seeds 2 Tbsp peanut butter
Fats and oils	1 tsp soft margarine 1 Tbsp low-fat mayonnaise 2 Tbsp light salad dressing 1 tsp vegetable oil

Avoid Calorie Creep

Many of us enjoy restaurants that provide large portions. We feel like we are getting good value for our money. However, most of us tend to eat more when we are served large portions. Even when you know you are full, it is easy to add several extra bites of dinner while waiting for others to finish. Here are several tricks for avoiding overeating in restaurants. (Much of this section is a summary of information that you will find in more detail in Chapters 2 and 4, but the advice warrants repeating.)

1. Choose the portion that you would like to eat, then bag the rest. Some people find it easier to ask the restaurant to wrap half of the meal before it comes to the table. Others put the excess food on the bread plate before eating. If you don't want to call attention to your method, mentally choose the portion that you want, and plan to stop when you have reached it.

2. Split entrées with your spouse or a friend. Surprisingly, most of these "half-portions" look like normal serving sizes. See how we have been tricked?

3. Split larger salads.

4. Choose an appetizer-sized portion for your main course.

5. Watch out for pasta meals. Very often the serving size is four to six times your target serving size. Eating half would still put you way over your calorie goals.

6. Ask restaurants to omit cheese and bacon toppings on salads, or ask to have them on the side, and then eat only a tiny portion.

7. Choose "slippery" dressings like vinaigrette or oil and vinegar. Less salad dressing is needed and much of it ends up on the plate.

8. Ask the waiter not to bring the bread until the salad course arrives. It is easy to mindlessly overeat bread

before dinner, when you are sitting in a restaurant filled with the smell of good food.

9   Spend more time paying attention to the dinner conversation and looking at your dinner companions rather than at the food. You may find that you forget to eat as much.

10. Split desserts. Some national chains have dessert portions sizes that can easily feed six and still leave everyone satisfied.

Lose Fat, Not Muscle

Muscle is our energy-burning powerhouse. Fat just goes along for the ride, storing up extra calories. As you lose weight, you want to maintain or increase your muscle tissue, and get rid of extra fat. Fast weight loss often causes people to lose muscle, which slows their metabolism. This usually leads to even quicker weight regain.

A balanced eating plan with adequate protein and plenty of dairy calcium will help you reach your goals and maintain your weight, fitness, and health. If you want to maintain muscle, clearly exercise needs to be a part of your healthy weight loss plan. Chapter 6 will help you with exercise plans that boost your muscle power and burn off fat.

Plan, Plan, Plan

Planning to succeed really does pay off.

1.   Make sure you keep all the right foods on hand. Stock up on the key DASH foods when you grocery shop. Buy more than you think you need.

2.   Take key DASH diet foods (fruits, raw veggies, dairy) to work for your lunches and snacks. Stock your mini fridge at the office, or bring an insulated bag with all the right foods.

3. Plan to include key DASH foods in your afternoon snacks.

4. Hit the salad bar for cut up fresh veggies and fruits.

5. Buy low-fat cheese that is individually packaged. Examples are Kraft® 2% Singles™, light string cheese, light Mini Baby Bel® cheese, and Laughing Cow® Light Spreadable cheese.

6. Buy lots of nonfat, artificially sweetened yogurt in many flavors.

7. Buy frozen vegetables in mass quantities. (I often buy five to ten packages at a time, for a two-person household.)

8. Do not skip meals or snacks. Satisfy your hunger while it is manageable.

9. Plan what you will eat for each meal and snack, each day.

10. Plan what you will eat before you go to a restaurant.

11. Remember your goal. Then plan to succeed.

Plan to have healthy choices available. If you consistently have trouble getting enough servings of some of the DASH food groups, add them to your snacks. Yogurt, light string cheese, and even a carton of skim milk are satisfying dairy foods that are excellent for snacks. Add some fresh fruit or a handful of nuts. Chomp on some cut up vegetables. Many people fall off track in mid to late afternoon, and hit the vending machines for candy, chips, or pop. Plan to have an afternoon snack and make sure you have healthy choices on hand.

Pay special attention to dairy foods. Try to include three to four servings each day. Dairy foods have been shown to help you become leaner, which is the goal of weight loss. Make sure that the overwhelming majority of your dairy is low-fat or nonfat.

When you are going out to dinner, think about what you will

order. Check out Appendix A for a list of lean meats. Plan on adding some vegetables. Even if you are just going out for a burger, plan to order a salad and a side of steamed vegetables. (And plan to eat only half the burger, since most restaurant portions tend to be large.) Add an extra vegetable-rich dish at Chinese restaurants or ask for a side dish of steamed vegetables. Limit your rice to one large spoonful, and use the steamed vegetables as the base for the rest of your meal. If you are going to splurge at night and have some less than healthy foods, stick to fruits, vegetables, and nonfat dairy at lunch, and try to limit the dinner portion size. Skip bread at dinner, and taste someone else's appetizer (without ordering one for yourself). A shared dessert will help keep the calories under control.

Focus on filling up with the DASH diet foods, and weight loss will be much simpler than you think.

DASHboard

1. Use the BMI table to find your healthy weight range.
2. Calculate your calorie needs.
3. Take special care to avoid "portion distortion."
4. Lose fat—not muscle. Add exercise to your routine, and get adequate protein in your diet.
5. Stock up and fill up on lower calorie DASH diet foods.

Tracking my Personal DASH Diet Action Plan

My current weight_____

My goal weight _____

My target calories _____

My two biggest calorie challenges are _____

_____

_____

I will avoid these by _____

_____

_____

What will keep me motivated? _____

_____

_____

_____

CHAPTER 6

EXERCISE YOUR RIGHT TO
LOWER BLOOD PRESSURE

Exercise is an important tool to help you lower your blood pressure. It also can improve cardiovascular health, reducing the risk of heart disease. It can also reduce your risk of certain types of cancer. Beyond all the health benefits, exercise makes you feel younger.

Most of my clients find that their energy level is much higher within the first month of starting an exercise program. There is energy in their step and they feel great. Exercise also helps improve mood, may relieve some symptoms of depression, and is a great stress-reliever.

So, why aren't we all already exercising? Many of us have very sedentary jobs, which we balance with more inactivity at home. Running around happens in the car, not by foot.

What are the special advantages of exercise for people with hypertension? Improved cardiovascular fitness can provide significant reductions in both systolic and diastolic blood pressure. Other heart disease risk factors can be reduced, such as obesity, the ratio of bad and good cholesterol, and the risk of developing type 2 diabetes. All of these heart disease risk factors are more common in people with hypertension than they are in the general population. People who are more fit have lower death rates than unfit people with normal blood pressure. Exercise has the potential to have striking benefits for improving the long-term health of people with high blood pressure.

How Much Exercise Do I Need?

People who have sedentary jobs may find that they need to exercise one hour each day just to keep even with the activity level of other people. This doesn't seem fair. However, many people with sedentary lives find that their total steps each day, as measured by a pedometer, are very low.

Does this apply to you? Take the pedometer challenge. Buy a pedometer (not the least expensive, it may not work properly or it may break quickly). Wear the pedometer all day. The average American takes five thousand steps per day. If your number is much lower than this, you may need to schedule longer exercise sessions. The goal is to take at least ten thousand steps daily. The pedometer is an excellent tool to provide instant feedback on your activity level. And it helps you track your progress in adding small changes into your routine.

These small changes can have a big payoff in increasing your overall activity level and burning more calories. Look at the following easy-to-make changes that will increase your activity without requiring extra time or special equipment. (And, yes, you may have heard several of these suggestions before—but, are you doing them?)

1. Park your car further away in the parking lot. In addition to saving your doors from dings, you add extra steps to your day, and save time by not driving around in circles looking for a closer parking space. Do this at the mall, the grocery store, and at work. If you drive to work in a large city, find a parking garage that is further from your office.

2. Take the train, bus, or subway to work. Each of these public transportation choices will provide you with extra walking time every weekday. They also can reduce stress, since you don't have to fight traffic to get to work. Read the paper, prepare for that presentation you have to make. Riding public transportation makes useful "found time."

3. If you live in a small town, ride your bike to work for a real exercise boost.

4. Climb the stairs. Walk up one floor and down two floors. As you become more fit, walk up two or more floors, and down at least five flights. At the office, use the bathrooms on a higher floor, and walk up and down. At home, don't make piles near the stairs to be taken up or down later. Take things upstairs (or downstairs) each time you find something that needs to be in another spot.

5. When you get to work, do some extra walking. Walk around the block once before going in. Walk to the opposite side of the building and then walk to your workplace.

6. Walk at lunch. Spend at least fifteen minutes walking during your lunch break. It will rev you up for the rest of the day and banish the mid-day droops.

Caution: Before starting an exercise program, people with hypertension should consult with their physicians regarding their fitness for an exercise program, and any restrictions. Many universities with exercise physiology programs have the capability of doing extensive evaluations of fitness levels, and designing exercise programs that are appropriate to improve overall fitness.

Exercise Guidelines

The American College of Sports Medicine (ACSM) is the leading group of practitioners that researches and makes recommendations for exercise guidelines for Americans. The suggestions in this section are based on position papers of the ACSM.

Exercise guidelines are generally based on three principles: frequency, intensity, and duration. Your routine should be designed to improve cardiovascular fitness, muscle strength, flexibility, and balance—all of which contribute to a better quality of life.

Exercise Benefits

Exercise will help you see improvements in the following areas:

♥ balance
♥ strengthened bones
♥ reduced body fat
♥ increased muscle mass
♥ improved digestive function
♥ metabolism boost
♥ lower mortality rate
♥ ease of performing daily activities
♥ improved lipid profiles (lower cholesterol, LDL, and triglycerides, and higher HDL)
♥ improved cardiac efficiency
♥ lower resting heart rate
♥ lower blood pressure
♥ increased joint mobility
♥ increased self-confidence

- ♥ reduced feeling of pain
- ♥ prevention of or decrease in symptoms of depression
- ♥ improved ability to manage stress
- ♥ increased intellectual function

Exercise Recommendations

It is recommended that adults adopt a well-balanced exercise regimen that includes aerobic activity, strength-building exercise, stretching and balance exercises.

RESISTANCE EXERCISE

Resistance exercise is also known as strength training, and helps boost metabolism, making it easier to reach and maintain a healthy weight. You can participate in strength training at a gym or health club, your local senior center, or at home. At the end of this chapter is a listing of books and other resources to help you design your resistance exercise program.

People with high blood pressure may be more likely to develop overly high blood pressure while doing resistance (strength) exercises. If you are planning an intensive strength training regimen, check with your physician regarding his or her recommendations for maximum diastolic blood pressure after exercise. Check your blood pressure immediately after each resistance exercise. If your diastolic blood pressure is higher than recommended, you may need to exercise with less resistance (less weight). You should also inform your physician about your response to the exercise.

ENDURANCE EXERCISE

Endurance exercise is also known as aerobic, cardiovascular, or cardio-respiratory activity. It can lower systolic and diastolic blood pressure about ten points. You don't have to overdo it, since moderate intensity exercise may be more beneficial than high intensity exercise. And it is helpful to start slowly and then increase intensity as your endurance improves. Aerobic activity includes walking, running, biking, dancing, hiking, and more. It will improve your cardiovascular fitness and help to reduce body fat, especially around your middle.

Your goal is to try to include at least thirty minutes of aerobic activity most days of the week. If you find it difficult to find a thirty-minute time slot, then break it into three ten-minute sessions.

FLEXIBILITY EXERCISE

Flexibility exercise is also known as stretching. Stretching has the ability to provide immediate benefits in your well-being. It can reduce the pain of arthritis, help prevent and speed recovery from injuries, and can help in preventing falls. Joints get nourishment from the surrounding fluid when they are alternately flexed and then relaxed, so stretching may help you feel less stiff and achy—and younger.

BALANCE EXERCISE

Preventing falls is a major objective as we get older. Many types of exercise can improve balance, such as yoga, Tai Chi, and other simple exercises. Some books and other resources with easy-to-perform balance exercises are shown at the end of this chapter.

Basic Exercise Guidelines

A basic exercise routine includes each of the exercise types: aerobic, resistance, flexibility, and balance, each week. Try to do aerobic, stretching, and balance exercise most days, and add some kind of resistance exercise two to three days per week (with at least one day in between sessions).

Plan to exercise each day. If you plan to exercise seven days a week, you are more likely to exercise at least five days, if something comes up on a couple of days. If you plan to exercise five days a

Judging Aerobic Exercise Intensity

Moderate Intensity—you can talk with ease.

High Intensity—it is difficult to talk or say more than a few words at a time.

week, schedule conflicts are likely to reduce it to only three days.

Plan to exercise 60 minutes each day if you are trying to lose weight. Weight maintainers may be able to get by with only 30 minutes per day.

Stay hydrated while you exercise. Consume 8 to 16 ounces of water before aerobic exercise, and 4 to 8 ounces every 15 to 20 minutes during exercise. Most people with high blood pressure need to avoid sports drinks, which can be high in salt and add extra calories. After exercising, include both carbs and protein in your snack or meal.

Exercise—How to Fit It In, How to Stick With It

Since many of us do not exercise enough—or at all—it requires concerted effort to make exercise a part of your daily routine. You need to choose exercise that you will enjoy and then make it easy for you to participate.

For many people, exercise is more likely to fit into their schedule if they can do it at home. This saves a lot of time. You don't have to drive anywhere, and you don't have to bring a bag with your clothes and other equipment (and probably forget some critical item). Whether you exercise first thing in the morning or in the evening, exercising at home, is more likely to get accomplished. Home equipment can include a treadmill, exercise bike, elliptical trainer, or weight machines. Exercising at home can be as simple as walking or running in your neighborhood or in a local park, or dancing to music in your living room.

Jump ropes, bikes, mini-tramps, roller blades, and free weights are all very inexpensive home exercise equipment.

It is important to choose a type of exercise you enjoy. You may think you don't enjoy any exercise. If so, you will benefit from finding something to do while you exercise to make it more enjoyable. Many people enjoy listening to music and books on tape; or watching movies, the news, or a favorite show. Find activities that will keep you engaged during your exercise routine. For example, morning news shows tend to have very short segments. In my experience (and that of many of my clients), this can cause you to focus more on the time, and seems to make the exercise drag on and on. National Public Radio might be a better choice to accompany your exercise, since its segments run longer, keeping you more interested. If you don't like to exercise, you need something to provide entertaining distraction during your entire exercise routine.

Personality is also an important consideration when making your exercise choices. Some people like to exercise in groups, and find it motivating. Health clubs, YMCAs, senior centers, and park districts all provide great exercise opportunities for people who like group exercise. Shop carefully for an exercise club where you feel comfortable. Being at a club with lots of people in spandex could inspire you to exercise harder, or it could make you reluctant to even show up. Some overweight women may feel more comfortable at female-only clubs. Many people like team sports, such as softball or basketball, or competitive individual sports such as golf or tennis.

If you find it hard to self-motivate, you may want to set up a session with a personal trainer, either at a club or at your home. Or find a friend who likes to do the same thing as you do, if you respond to peer pressure.

Exercise can improve your balance, make you stronger, and improve your stamina. Exercise will help you feel younger. The point is: find something that suits your time needs, personality, fitness level, and body comfort level. And then, do it!

Following are many great ideas for adding active time to your life:

walking	jogging	running
triathlons	body building	long-distance running
inline skating	frisbee	stretching
gardening	yoga	t'ai-chi
karate	swimming	ballet
rowing	ice-skating	running on treadmill
canoeing	kayaking	walking/hiking clubs
circuit training	weight training	Pilates
exercise ball	free weights	mini-trampoline
aerobics	aerobic dance	jazz dance
square dancing	belly dancing	ballroom dancing
folk dancing	hiking	mountain biking
cycling	curling	skiing
mountaineering	jumping rope	basketball
softball	racquetball	handball
golf	hockey	tennis
calisthenics	stationary bike	stepper
elliptical machine	synchronized swimming	

Getting Started

How do you get on track with your exercise routine? You may need to get exercise clothes and shoes, some home exercise equipment, and find a gym or other place to work out. Set the stage for success by breaking down the barriers.

Make sure you get good shoes for the type of activity you plan to do. Gym shoes should provide good support for your foot and your walking style. If you find it difficult to bend over and tie your shoes, try to find slip-on gym shoes.

If it fits into your budget and into your living space, invest in good quality exercise equipment. A home treadmill, elliptical trainer, stationary bike, cross-country ski machine, or other aerobic equipment will make it easy to exercise in all weather conditions. Free weights allow you to become stronger. Exercise balls, bands, ramps and more can increase the fun and decrease boredom. EBay or second hand stores can be inexpensive sources for home equipment.

Burn a CD with your favorite tunes for your walking or running program. Get a book on tape from your local library. Get a portable radio, CD or MP3 player, or cassette deck. Put a TV and a DVD player in front of your treadmill, or set up a boom box with a remote control to pump up the volume as you exercise harder. Find something to make the time you spend exercising more enjoyable.

Make your plan for your exercise routine. When will you exercise? Where will it happen? Lay out your exercise clothes the night before, to help get you started and remove another barrier.

WHERE?

Many people find that it is difficult to make the time to exercise. If you can exercise at home, you may cut down on the time you need to exercise. Taking a walk early in the morning means only one shower and no travel time to the gym. Use your home exercise equipment or enjoy walking in your neighborhood, a local mall, park district facility, school track, or gym. Paying for a gym membership may motivate you to exercise, so as not to waste your money. There are many locales for exercise.

WHEN?

Studies have shown that people are more likely to stick with their exercise plan if they exercise early in the morning. Daily life issues are less likely to intrude on your early morning routine. I personally like to exercise first thing, since I am not awake enough to notice that I don't like to exercise. You may find that you can fit in exercise at lunch time at work. Or, put dinner in the oven and hit the treadmill to de-stress after your day. Or perhaps, evenings after the kids go to bed will be "your time." If you do strength training at home, you may find it easy to do while you are watching your favorite television show.

Exercise and Anti-Hypertensive Medications

Some medications for hypertension can alter your response to exercise. Please check with your physician for any cautions about the type of exercise you can perform.

Exercise Resources

BOOKS (Note: you can often find less expensive copies through online booksellers, even for out-of-print books.)

Strong Women Stay Young, Miriam Nelson, Bantam Books, 1997

Strong Women Stay Slim, Miriam Nelson, Bantam Books, 1999

Exercise: A Guide from the National Institute on Aging, National Institute on Aging.

Stretching, 20th Anniversary Edition, Bob and Jean Anderson, Shelter Publications, 2000

MAGAZINES

Shape

Self

Fitness

Prevention

WEBSITES

http://nihseniorhealth.gov/exercise/toc.html *Many resources, free books, and an exercise video for seniors.*

http://www.cdc.gov/nccdphp/dnpa/physical/index.htm *Physical fitness resources from the Centers on Disease Control and Prevention.*

http://www.collagevideo.com *Online catalogue of exercise videos.*

http://dynamixmusic.com *CDs to energize your exercise routine.*

For more current resources, visit our Website at: http://DASHdiet.org/exercise.asp

DASHboard

1. Plan to exercise each day.
2. Plan for a mix of aerobic, strength, flexibility, and balance exercises.
3. You may need to exercise 60 minutes per day if you are trying to lose weight.
4. Do exercise that you enjoy. You are more likely to keep going.
5. Morning exercise may help avoid schedule conflicts.
6. Consider your personality type when choosing your exercise program.
7. Exercising at home may fit a hectic schedule.
8. Invest in your health. Buy equipment that allows you to exercise at home.
9. Stay hydrated while you exercise.
10. Even small bouts of exercise can have health benefits.

Tracking my Personal DASH Diet Action Plan

What exercises will I incorporate into my routine, how long, and how often?

_____, _____ minutes, ____ x/week

_____, _____ minutes, ____ x/week

_____, _____ minutes, ____ x/week

Where will I do these exercises? _____

_____

What time of day will I exercise? _____

_____

_____

What equipment do I need? _____

_____

_____

Additional activities I enjoy: _____

_____

_____

What will keep me motivated? _____

_____

_____

_____

CHAPTER 7

OTHER HEALTH CONCERNS

People with high blood pressure often have other health concerns. They may have type 2 diabetes or metabolic syndrome. Hypertension is associated with increased risk of other cardiovascular diseases, such as atherosclerosis, congestive heart failure, stroke, and coronary artery disease. Fortunately the DASH diet can improve the health of most people with these conditions.

Diabetes

If you have type 1 diabetes (also known as insulin-dependent or juvenile diabetes) you should consult with a registered dietitian before making any changes in your diet. You need to be sure that you are coordinating your food intake with your insulin and your activity.

People who have type 2 diabetes (also known as non-insulin dependent or adult-onset diabetes) can usually follow the DASH diet and improve their blood sugar control. The high fiber intake can result in lower blood sugar. Some of the key minerals found in the DASH foods may be associated with improved sensitivity to insulin. This can reduce the need for medication or supplemental insulin and slow the progression of the disease. All of the key DASH foods are beneficial for people with diabetes. Whole grains, fruits, vegetables, low-fat and nonfat dairy, and even nuts are known to have special benefits for improving health for people with diabetes. Many dietitians have found that nuts improve glucose control in people with diabetes. The fiber in whole grains, fruits and vegetables can slow the absorption of sugar, avoiding large swings in blood glucose. Fruits and vegetables are rich in antioxidants, which may be associated with reduction in complications from diabetes. Choosing low-fat or nonfat dairy, lean meats and poultry help reduce the risk of developing high cholesterol. This is an important benefit, since people with diabetes are at higher risk for heart disease. Weight loss and exercise have been shown to reduce the risk of developing type 2 diabetes or to reverse mild diabetes. The entire DASH Diet Action Plan supports good health, even with diabetes.

Metabolic Syndrome

Dietary advice gets more complicated when high blood pressure gets mixed up with high triglycerides or elevated blood sugars. This gets into territory that may be diagnosed as Metabolic Syndrome or Syndrome X. (A syndrome, unlike a disease, involves a condition where not all of the symptoms are required for diagnosis.) A hallmark of metabolic syndrome is insulin resistance or the inability to properly utilize insulin. People with insulin resistance may have their symptoms worsened by a high-refined carbohydrate, low-fat diet.

Insulin resistance is a condition where the body does not respond well to the insulin produced by the body. Blood sugars remain elevated longer than normal after a meal. To compensate, the body pumps out extra insulin in an attempt to lower the blood sugar. The extra insulin induces the body to produce more cholesterol, and also plumps up fat cells (especially in our abdomen). Instead of storing sugar in our muscles for quick energy, we store the sugar in our fat cells where it is converted into fat. Our liver also tries to clean up extra blood sugar by converting it into triglycerides (more fat). Our body packages the triglycerides into vehicles that soak up cholesterol from the HDL (good cholesterol). This shrinks the HDL, reducing its ability to clean up cholesterol in the arteries and increasing the risk of heart disease.

Diagnosis of Metabolic Syndrome

Three or more of the following:

♥ Waist circumference greater than 40 inches for men or 35 inches for women.

♥ Triglycerides higher than 150.

♥ HDL < 40 for men or <50 for women.

♥ Blood pressure higher than 130/85 without medication.

♥ Fasting glucose greater than 100.

Insulin resistance may progress to a condition called "pre-diabetes," which is when the fasting blood sugar (glucose) measurement is between 100 and 125. People with metabolic syndrome will typically have blood sugars above 85. Although still in the normal range, it is higher than optimal fasting blood sugar, which is 70 to 85. Having a fasting blood sugar higher than 85 may indicate that you are not responding as well to insulin. Your triglycerides may also be elevated. When the body has had to produce extra insulin for several years, eventually it wears out its ability to produce enough insulin. Then the person will develop type 2 diabetes. The body cannot produce enough insulin to keep blood sugar under control.

DASH Diet Adjustments with Metabolic Syndrome or Type 2 Diabetes

Avoiding high amounts of refined carbohydrates can support better glucose control in people with type 2 diabetes or metabolic syndrome. You can still include all of the key DASH foods, such as fruits, vegetables, low-fat dairy, nuts, beans, and lean meats. However, having piles of pasta, white rice, bagels, and pretzels may not be so helpful.

What are refined carbohydrates? Any of the white grain foods are considered to be refined. They generally are very low in fiber, and low in minerals that are associated with improved blood pressure control. Refined grains include refined flour, white rice, and all the foods that are made from them. Bagels, pasta, pretzels, sweetened cereals, Italian bread, French bread, pastries, cakes, and cookies all contain refined carbohydrates. Whole grains include whole wheat, brown rice, rye, oats, and pumpernickel. Although these grains are all brown, not all brown grain foods are made from 100% whole grains. Sometimes the brown color comes from caramel food coloring. And some breads and cereals have labels that say they contain whole grains, but they may have only a small amount. If you want whole grains, it is important to check the food labels to be sure that all the flour in a bread or cereal comes from 100% whole grains.

All starches, from refined and whole grains, are broken down into glucose (the sugar in blood sugar measurements) during digestion. Therefore, both starch and sugar can elevate blood sugar. Even though starch is considered to be a complex carbohydrate, it does turn into glucose, and it happens relatively quickly with refined carbohydrates. So, the question is not whether you should choose simple carbs or complex carbs, but rather, how can you include more high-fiber carbs.

Foods that have more fiber tend to be broken down and absorbed more slowly than refined carbohydrates. This will result in less demand for the body to pump out extra insulin to keep blood sugar under control. This is certainly a nice benefit for people with type 2 diabetes or metabolic syndrome.

A lower (moderate) carbohydrate diet may be beneficial for weight reduction for people with insulin resistance. If refined carbohydrates are limited, it will make it easier to include more servings of fruits, vegetables, and dairy foods. Key DASH nutrients, such as calcium, potassium, magnesium, and fiber are not found in appreciable quantities in refined carbohydrates.

The DASH Diet Action Plan also includes recommendations for weight loss and exercise. Research has shown that these steps can help reverse or delay the onset of pre-diabetes or type 2 diabetes better than medication. And research has shown that people who include more whole grains and dairy in their diets, as recommended in the DASH eating plan, are less likely to develop type 2 diabetes.

Artery-Blocking High Cholesterol

The DASH diet has been shown to lower cholesterol. Cholesterol in the blood is found in several different forms. HDL (high density lipoprotein) is the good form of cholesterol. It is a form of "packaging" for cholesterol that actually cleans up the cholesterol in arteries. The LDL (low density lipoprotein) is the cholesterol package that tends to deposit cholesterol in the arteries. In general, we like to have more of the good cholesterol (HDL) and less of the bad cholesterol (LDL). Diet, weight reduction, and exercise as promoted in the DASH Diet Action Plan will support improving cholesterol profiles.

Specific nutrition recommendations for lowering cholesterol

include: limited intake of dietary cholesterol, saturated and trans fats (discussed in Chapter 9), and increased intake of soluble fiber, soy foods, and plant stanols. The strategies are to reduce intake of the raw materials for making cholesterol (saturated and trans fats) and to reduce absorption of cholesterol and its raw materials. The DASH diet helps with both.

We want to reduce intake of these fats. The DASH diet encourages the use of low-fat or nonfat dairy foods, and lean meats, fish, and poultry, all of which help provide an eating plan low in saturated fats. The DASH diet is low in trans fats, since there is not much room for the empty calorie snacks and desserts that are often big sources of trans fats. Sources of heart healthy fats in the DASH diet include olive

Classifications of Blood Lipid Levels

Total Cholesterol
Desirable . . . . <200
Borderline high 200-239
High . . . . 240+

LDL Cholesterol
Desirable with CVD . . . . <70
Optimal . . . . <100
Near or above optimal. . . . 100-129
Borderline high 130-159
High 160-189
Very high . . . . 190+

HDL Cholesterol
Low . . . . <40
High (desirable) . . . . 60+

Triglycerides (triacylglyerols)
Normal. . . . . <150
Borderline high 150-199
High 200-499
Very high . . . . 500+

oil, avocados, nuts, fatty fish, as well as corn, soy and other vegetable oils.

The high fiber in the DASH diet helps to lower cholesterol by reducing absorption of cholesterol and fats. Fiber that is especially good for helping to lower cholesterol is called functional fiber or soluble fiber. Some well-known examples include the beta-glucan in oats, pectin in apples, and psyllium found in

Metamucil™. Most fruits and vegetables contain fiber that will help to lower cholesterol. You can find a list of some of these key foods in Chapter 9.

Another dietary change that supports lowering cholesterol is adding plant stanols/sterols, which are found in some margarines, including Benecol™ and Take Control™, and some fruit juices. Research has shown that they can help lower cholesterol by up to 14%. Soy protein (and the fiber found in many soy products) can support lowering cholesterol as well.

We want HDL cholesterol to be high. Having HDL greater than 60 is considered to remove one risk factor for heart disease. Lifestyle changes that will improve HDL include: stop smoking, add exercise, and avoid a diet high in refined carbs.

DASHboard

Metabolic Syndrome, Type 2 Diabetes

1. Avoid high-carb, low-fat diets. Choose moderate carb, moderate protein, moderate fat.
2. Add more fiber to your diet, from key DASH diet foods: whole grains, beans, nuts, vegetables, and fruits.
3. Include three or four servings of low-fat or nonfat dairy each day.
4. Add aerobic exercise to help burn off belly fat.
5. Add strength exercise to reduce insulin resistance.
6. Limit saturated fat and trans fat intake.

High Cholesterol

1. Limit intake of saturated fats, trans fats, and dietary cholesterol. Keep fat intake moderate.
2. Include foods rich in soluble fiber.
3. Stop smoking, increase exercise, and avoid overdoing refined carbs to increase HDL.

Tracking my Personal DASH Diet Action Plan

	Current	Target
Fasting glucose:	_____	_____
Cholesterol	_____	_____
HDL	_____	_____
LDL	_____	_____
Triglycerides:	_____	_____

Changes I will make that will improve my blood glucose control:

_____

_____

_____

_____

Changes I will make to lower my cholesterol and/or triglycerides: _____

_____

_____

_____

_____

I will increase HDL by making these changes: _____

_____

_____

_____

_____

_____

CHAPTER 8

LIFESTYLE CHANGES TO HELP LOWER BLOOD PRESSURE

In this book we focus on healthy diet, weight loss, and exercise as lifestyle changes that help lower blood pressure. Additional key lifestyle changes that will help support lowering your blood pressure include smoking cessation and limiting alcohol consumption.

Alcohol

Healthy alcohol consumption is no more than one drink per day for women, and two drinks for men. In addition to raising blood pressure, alcohol is a source of empty calories that can make it difficult to lose weight. Alcohol can cause elevated triglycerides, which is another heart disease risk.

Many people over-consume alcohol in social settings. A good party strategy can be to alternate alcohol with water or other nonalcoholic beverages. That way you still have a drink in your hand, but you aren't drinking alcohol.

What counts as a drink?

- ♥ 12 ounces of beer
- ♥ 5 ounces of wine
- ♥ 1 ounce of 80-proof whiskey, rum, vodka

Smoking

Smoking creates conditions that make it easier for cholesterol to stick onto the lining of the arteries, facilitating the blockage of arteries. In case you need a reminder, the National Institutes of Health list the following reasons for quitting smoking:

- ♥ Reduce the risk of having a heart attack or stroke.
- ♥ Reduce the risk of getting lung cancer, emphysema, and other lung diseases.
- ♥ Be able to climb stairs and walk without getting out of breath.
- ♥ Have younger skin, with fewer wrinkles.
- ♥ Eliminate morning cough.
- ♥ Reduce the number of coughs, colds, and earaches your child will have.
- ♥ Have more energy to pursue physical activities you enjoy.

Within twenty minutes of your last cigarette, your blood pressure and pulse decrease. Within eight hours, the carbon monoxide level in your blood normalizes. After ten years, your risk of dying from lung cancer is almost the same as for someone who has never smoked. After fifteen years of not smoking, your risk of a stroke or heart disease is the same as for a lifelong non-smoker.

Decide today that you no longer want to be a smoker.

DASHboard

1. If you drink alcohol, do so in moderation. Limit to no more than one drink per day for women, two for men.
2. Stop smoking.

Tracking my Personal DASH Diet Action Plan

I will limit myself to _____ drinks per day.

I will not start (or restart smoking) _____ yes _____ no.

I will quit smoking _____ yes _____ no by doing _____

_____

by (date) _____.

CHAPTER 9

A HEALTHY MIX OF FATS, PROTEINS, AND CARBS

Since the late 1980s, the American public has been hearing the message that dietary fat is bad. We were told to reduce the fat in our diet. They said that lowering fat would reduce our caloric intake and reduce our risk of heart disease and cancer. Companies rushed to produce fat-free products to meet the new consumer demand.

Consumers feasted on SnackWell™ cookies, bagels, and pretzels, low-fat foods that were assumed to be healthier and to have less calories than the Oreos™, doughnuts, and Doritos™ they replaced. We heard that Americans were eating too much meat, so we cut down or eliminated meat altogether. We were told that a high-carb diet was the key to a healthier diet and would control weight.

The percentage of fat calories in the American diet decreased—we consumed less protein and more carbs—yet Americans became fatter.

Where Did We Get Off Track?

The truth about fat is much more complicated than just having less of it in our diets. While we were eliminating fats, we may have eliminated too much protein or may have overdone refined carbs. Getting on track with a healthy diet means re-establishing a balance of fats, protein, and carbs, and choosing healthy fats and carbs that are fiber-rich.

Choosing food that tastes great and is satisfying can help us eat less, while enjoying it more. Many low-fat or low-carb foods simply don't taste very good, and many have about the same calories as the foods they replace. Compared with high-carb meals, moderate amounts of fat and protein help to provide satiety, improve flavor, and help us avoid overeating.

There are healthy fats that we want to include in our diets, and fats that we definitely need to limit. We want to make sure to get enough protein and fiber in our diets. The DASH diet supports this, and shows that these dietary changes help to lower blood pressure, reduce cholesterol, and provide a foundation for weight loss.

In this chapter you will learn which fats are healthy, what foods are good sources of these healthy fats, what foods are lean and protein-rich, and how to choose carbs that are rich in more than just calories, and won't cause your blood sugar to soar.

Healthy Fats

All naturally occurring fats are mixtures. They contain fatty acids with different chain lengths, different amounts of saturation, and differing health effects. Some fats are essential, which means that we have to get them in our diets, in the right amounts. Some fats can make us healthier, while others can increase our risks for many diseases, especially heart disease.

Based on current knowledge, the especially healthy fats include monounsaturated fats (olives, avocados, nuts) and omega-3 fatty acids (fish oils), while saturated fats are considered to be associated with increased risk for heart disease. Polyunsaturated fats fit in the middle, having some health promoting properties and some potential risk.

SATURATED VERSUS UNSATURATED FATS

One of the main classifications of fats has two categories, those that are saturated and those that are unsaturated. The unsaturated fats are further divided into monounsaturated and polyunsaturated fats. Saturation refers to whether or not there is a full complement of hydrogen on the fat. Saturated fats (SFAs) have all the hydrogen they can possibly have; that is, they are "saturated" with hydrogen. Monounsaturated fats (MUFAs) are missing hydrogen in one spot, and polyunsaturated fats (PUFAs) are missing hydrogen in two or more spots. The PUFAs can be further divided as to where the unsaturation points occur, such as omega-3 and omega-6 fatty acids.

The MUFAs and PUFAs are liquids, while most saturated fats are solid at room temperature. In order to turn liquid fats, such as corn or soybean oil, into solid fats to make margarine or shortening, the oil has to be hydrogenated. This makes the fat more saturated. The process of hydrogenating the oils can create trans fatty acids, which are considered to increase the risk of heart disease.

In general, most saturated fats, including trans fatty acids, are associated with increased risk of developing high blood cholesterol. Guidelines for healthy eating encourage people to get less saturated and hydrogenated fats in their diet. Monounsaturated fats are considered to be heart healthy and are encouraged in the diet. The omega-3 fatty acids are also especially heart healthy. The other polyunsaturated fats do not cause an elevation in cholesterol levels and so are also considered relatively heart-healthy.

The best recommendations are to keep fat at a moderate level (between 25 and 35 percent of total calories) by choosing lean meats, fish, and poultry; low-fat and nonfat dairy products (to reduce saturated fat intake); include fish in your diet a few times a week (to increase omega-3 fatty acids); include moderate amounts of oils rich in monounsaturated fats, as well as nuts and seeds; limit foods containing trans fats; and limit or avoid fried foods.

MORE ON FATS AND HEALTH

Both MUFAs and PUFAs help to lower cholesterol. MUFAs have an added benefit, since they do not lower the "good cholesterol," known as HDL. PUFAs can lower good cholesterol along with lowering bad cholesterol. PUFAs are also a little less stable and may be susceptible to oxidation, which is undesirable. We need to get enough of these essential fats, but we don't want to overdo it.

A special type of PUFAs are the omega-3 fatty acids, such as those found in fish oils (DHA and EPA). Studies have shown that people who consume more fatty fish or fish oil supplements are less likely to die from heart disease, and possibly are less likely to develop cancer. Other potential benefits from fish oils include reduced risk of developing diabetes, reduced triglycerides, reduced blood clotting tendencies, reduced depression, and reduced inflammation. Omega-3 fatty acids are also found in plant oils, such as flaxseed and walnuts, but current research suggests that little of these fatty acids are converted into the desirable DHA.

I am not recommending for or against taking fish oil supplements. Any supplementation should be discussed with your physician and a registered dietitian. If you are taking blood thinners, like warfarin (Coumadin) or Plavix, fish oil could make you more likely to develop a bleeding problem or be susceptible to a hemorrhagic stroke. Many other over-the-counter medications and supplements, such as aspirin, vitamin E, garlic, and ginkgo biloba, inhibit blood clotting, so adding fish oil supplements could increase the risk of bleeding problems or stroke. Some studies have shown a negative interaction of fish oil supplements with certain diabetic medications. If you want to use fish oil supplements, be sure to discuss it with your physician (and/or a registered dietitian).

FOOD SOURCES OF FATS

There are many reasons for including various types of fats in your diet. When choosing which fats to add to foods or choosing foods that naturally contain fats, you can consider taste, cost, stability to heat, and health effects.

SATURATED FATS

Animal foods, including beef, pork, and dairy products, are the largest source of saturated fats in the typical American diet. However, today the beef and pork industries produce leaner animals, and much leaner cuts of meat. Reduced-fat or nonfat dairy foods allow you to add calcium to your diet without overdoing saturated fat.

And, as the following chart shows, saturated fats do not come just from animal foods. Coconut oil and palm oil are high in saturated fats. After coconut oil, butterfat has the highest percentage of saturated fat, and butterfat is the fat found in all dairy that is not fat-free. You can make a big impact on your choles-

117

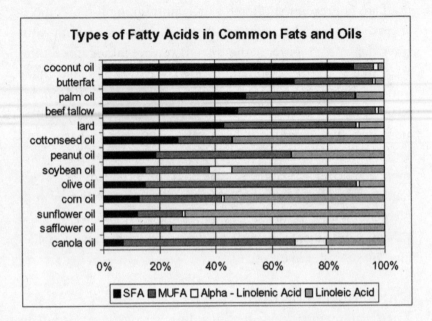

Types of Fatty Acids in Common Fats and Oils

terol by replacing full-fat dairy foods with nonfat or reduced fat products, such as nonfat frozen yogurt, reduced-fat cheese, nonfat cottage cheese, and skim milk.

It may be a surprise to many people that there are many types of beef and pork that are quite lean today and can be part of a heart healthy diet. These lean cuts are low in saturated fats, and have cholesterol content similar to skinless poultry. To help you select lean cuts, a detailed comparison of fat content and calories of various meats, fish, and poultry are listed in Appendix A.

MONOUNSATURATED FATS

Olive oil and canola oil are the best known sources of monoun-saturated fats. Olive oil contains slightly more MUFA than canola, but also contains slightly more SFA. Avocados, nuts and seeds and their oils are other good sources of MUFAs. If you like peanut butter, I recommend using the natural versions, which are not hydrogenated. Be sure to keep natural peanut butter in the refrigerator after opening, to avoid rancidity. And keep nut intake under control. A serving of nuts is just ¼ cup. One serving has the protein of 1 ounce of meat, and the calories of 3 ounces.

POLYUNSATURATED FATS

Soy and corn oil are the most popular sources of polyunsaturated fats. Safflower, cottonseed, and sunflower oil are other readily available sources of PUFAs. There is a new variety of safflower that is high in oleic acid, which is a MUFA, so you may soon see more safflower oil that is rich in MUFAs. The two essential fatty acids (necessary for health) are PUFAs (linolenic and linoleic acids).

High fat, but not as high calorie as you think . . .

Olives, 5 small . . . . . .20 Cal
Avocado, 1 oz. . . . . . .50 Cal

OMEGA-3 FATTY ACIDS

Omega-3 fats are a subset of the PUFAs. Flaxseed oil is the best known plant source; soy and walnuts are also good sources. The plant oils provide alpha-linolenic acid (ALA), which is an essential fatty acid. The body converts some ALA into DHA and EPA, which are found in cold-water fatty fish, and are the key health-promoting omega-3 fats. It is believed that only small amounts of ALA get turned into DHA, so fish remains the best source. (Please see Appendix B for a list of common fish sources and their omega-3 content.) Flaxseed and flaxseed oil are very susceptible to rancidity, so if you decide to use flax, be sure that it is stored in a cold, dark place, buy small quantities that you will use up relatively quickly, and if using flaxseed, grind just before using.

HYDROGENATED FATS

Shortening and margarine are two common sources of hydrogenated fats. In general, any vegetable oil that has been turned into a solid is hydrogenated, and may contain trans fats.

Food labels are a good source of information on hydrogenated fats in food. Look for the terms hydrogenated fats or partially-hydrogenated fats in the ingredient list. Most baked goods, such as snack crackers, pastries, and cookies are rich in these types of fats, since they are made with shortening. Many margarines and peanut butters are also sources of trans fats. Labeling for trans fatty acids is now included on the Nutrition Facts panel on packaged food so that you can better judge which foods are low in trans fats.

For example, many soft spread margarines are lower in trans fats than stick margarines. Since trans fats are now appearing on labels, many food products are being reformulated by manufacturers to have little or no trans fats. Use the Nutrition Facts label as your final word on whether or not foods with hydrogenated fats have the unhealthy trans fats.

Protein

Protein is a basic building block for the body. It forms the basis of muscles, skin, and organs. Specialized proteins act as hormones, while others act as enzymes to help digest and metabolize food. Proteins help to carry nutrients, such as fats and minerals, in the blood.

As seen in the diagram on the following page, even though carbs and protein can be converted into fat, and fat and protein into carbs; protein cannot be made from fat or carbohydrates. You have to be sure to get enough protein in your diet to maintain or build muscle, which will keep your metabolism high.

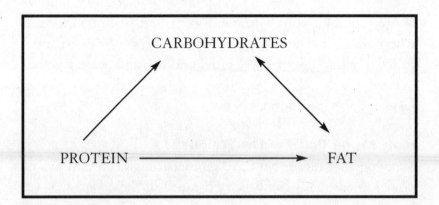

PROTEIN QUALITY

Amino acids are the building blocks of all proteins in our bodies. Some amino acids are essential, meaning that we have to obtain them from food, and some amino acids can be made in the body by transforming one of the essential amino acids into a nonessential one.

In general, animal proteins are better quality than vegetable protein. The quality is based on whether the protein has all of the essential amino acids in the right proportion. Fortunately for vegetarians, getting vegetable protein from a variety of sources improves the total protein quality of the diet. Many vegetable proteins are complementary to each other by filling in the gaps for inadequate amino acids from other foods.

Most animal proteins provide all of the essential amino acids in the right amounts. The proteins in eggs, dairy, meat, poultry, and fish are all high quality proteins. Isolated soy protein is considered to be a high quality plant protein. Other plant proteins, such as corn, wheat, and beans are incomplete proteins, but still are beneficial in a diet that is balanced with "complementary" proteins that are higher in the deficient amino acids. Some good examples of complementary plant proteins include rice and beans, corn and beans, wheat and corn, and peanut butter and wheat bread. It is interesting that many of these foods are often paired in ethnic cuisines. We often find rice and beans together in Caribbean and Latin American dishes, as well as in Chinese, Japanese, and Indian foods.

How Much Protein Do We Need?

Many popular diet books have promoted high consumption of protein foods. This conflicts with much of the advice that we have received over the past several decades, urging Americans to reduce the amount of protein in their diets. The DASH diet is a moderate plan that emphasizes adequate protein. Studies show that getting enough protein helps to lower blood pressure.

So then, how much do we need? The new Dietary Recommended Intake (DRI) says that protein should be 15 to 35% of your calories, or minimally 0.4 grams protein per pound of weight (or more accurately, 0.8 grams per kilogram).

The amount of protein that you need is proportional to your weight, so if you are on a weight loss plan, you will want to maintain (or possibly increase) your protein intake, while cutting empty carbs. A weight maintenance version of the DASH diet will probably provide about 20% of calories from protein. People who are on a DASH weight loss plan will have a higher percentage of total calories from protein.

What does this mean in real life terms? If you weigh 154 pounds, the minimum amount of protein that you would need is 56 grams. You can get 58 grams of protein by consuming two glasses of milk and six ounces of meat, fish, or poultry. If you add six servings of grains and four servings of vegetables, you will add another 26 grams of protein.

So, you can see that it isn't very difficult to get the amount of protein that you need in a day.

Protein Content of Foods

Food Group	Serving Size	Protein Grams
Grains	1 slice bread, ½ cup cooked grains, such as pasta or oatmeal, ½ English muffin or bun, ¼ bagel, 1/3 cup rice	3
Vegetables	½ cup cooked vegetables, 1 cup raw leafy greens	2
Nuts	1 oz. or ¼ cup	7
Beans	½ cup	7
Dairy	1 cup milk, 8 oz. yogurt, 1 oz. cheese	8
Meat	1 oz. meat, poultry or fish, 1 egg	7

FOOD SOURCES OF PROTEIN

Where do we find protein in our diet? Most of the food groups, except for fruits and fats, contain protein. Grains, vegetables, dairy foods, meats, fish, and poultry, along with eggs, legumes, nuts, and seeds all contain protein. The richest sources are meats, fish, poultry, and eggs. And, in general, animal sources of protein have the best quality, with grains having poor quality protein. The above list shows the amount of protein in different types of foods.

LOW-FAT AND LEAN PROTEIN-RICH FOODS

The best protein sources are low in saturated fats and rich in vitamins and minerals. They include lean meats, fish, poultry, low-fat and nonfat dairy foods, soy products, beans, nuts, and egg whites.

When the relationship of heart disease with cholesterol and high-fat animal foods was first noted, the prevailing wisdom told us to reduce our intake of red meat and most dairy foods. People eliminated or reduced their red meat consumption and cut dairy intake. But now, many of my clients tell me that they are tired of having "the same old chicken" for dinner every night, and most Americans have diets sadly lacking in dairy. The great news is that there are many healthy alternatives. There are a variety of lean meats, and low-fat and nonfat dairy foods available today. Healthy diets can include red meat and dairy foods that are low in fat, along with poultry, fish, and vegetable protein sources.

The key to leaner meats is to look for cuts that are called loin or round. Sirloin, tenderloin, and loin chops (including New York strip steaks) are all lean cuts. Another helpful tip is to choose meats that are graded "select." Prime and choice grades have more fat and calories. Fortunately, select is the grade that is available in most grocery stores. When you are in better restaurants you are more likely to find choice or prime meats. You may decide to order seafood if you want a lower fat restaurant choice. Prime rib is a very fatty beef choice, since it comes from beef that is graded prime. Beef tenderloin is a lower fat option and equally tender and flavorful.

Within each type of protein food group, there are likely to be many lean choices to keep you from getting bored with your meals. If you want to have beef, top loin chops and sirloin make good steak-type choices. You can make a burger with 95% lean ground sirloin, which is almost as lean as the same amount of white chicken meat. Pork is generally lean. Even ham is now a great low-fat choice. If you like the taste of barbecued ribs, try pork chops with barbecue sauce, for a meatier, lighter choice.

Skinless chicken and turkey breast make tasty low-fat choices. Surprisingly, much of the ground turkey in grocery stores contains added turkey fat and ground skin, and often has more fat than lean ground beef. Most fish and seafood is low in fat, with some being extremely low-fat. Expand your repertoire, and break out of your dinner-time rut with protein choices that won't contribute to a cholesterol problem.

Appendix A provides lists with many types of meat, poultry, and fish that will give you more lean choices at home and in restaurants. The tables provide calories, fat grams, saturated fat, and cholesterol content.

Reduced-fat dairy products also are terrific protein sources. These lower fat dairy foods give you a big payoff in lower calories and saturated fat. For example, skim milk (now called fat-free milk) only has 90 calories compared with 150 for whole milk (with 3.5% butterfat). Skim has just as much protein and calcium, without the fat.

Plant protein foods are often fat-free. Beans and grains have little or no fat. Since nuts and seeds are high-fat protein foods, it is helpful to watch your serving sizes. Nuts are rich in minerals, fiber, and monounsaturated fats, so there are substantial health benefits from including moderate amounts of nuts in your diet.

Fat content is not the only factor you should consider when making protein choices. Fatty cold-water fish are good sources of omega-3 fatty acids. Even though shrimp is high in cholesterol, it is very low in saturated fat and calories, and is considered to be heart healthy. Beef is very rich in minerals and vitamins. A 3-ounce serving of lean beef contains only 10% of the daily value (DV) for calories, but 50% of the protein, 39% of the zinc, 37% of the vitamin B12, 16% of vitamin B6, and 14% of the iron. Milk, yogurt, and cheese are all rich in calcium. Beans are rich in soluble fiber and contribute iron and zinc. Nuts and seeds contribute fiber, vitamin E, and minerals. Fat content is an important consideration, but don't make it your only cue. You have more good protein choices than you think.

The DASH Diet Action plan encourages you to include a variety of low-fat protein foods in your diet. Each day you should include about 6 ounces from the meat group (or plant protein) and 2 to 3 servings of low-fat dairy foods. And you should include 4 to 5 servings of nuts or beans each week.

Carbohydrates

What is all the talk about "bad" carbs and "good" carbs? In general, good carbs do not cause your blood sugar to shoot up, and they are usually rich sources of vitamins, minerals, and fiber. Bad carbs may provide empty calories, without bringing much nutritional value.

The concept of identifying how likely carbohydrate-rich foods are to cause blood sugar (glucose) to rise is called the glycemic index (GI). It is considered by many experts to be an important consideration for weight loss and for managing blood sugar. Simple sugars and starch are easy for the body to break down and absorb. Most starch gets digested to glucose, which is directly related to rises in glucose in the blood.

Foods that can cause blood sugar to rise quickly are identified as high glycemic index foods. Low GI foods tend to have high fiber content. People with high blood pressure may also be sensitive to high GI foods.

The DASH diet is rich in low GI carbs, loaded with fiber. When you eat 4 to 5 servings of fruits and 4 to 5 servings of vegetables each day, you automatically add lots of fiber to your diet. Whole grains are another great way to add fiber. And the DASH diet recommends 4 to 5 servings per week of nuts and beans, adding yet more fiber. The typical DASH diet plan, at 2,000 calories, contains over 31 grams of fiber.

126

Fiber

Fiber has additional benefits beyond helping to keep blood sugar on a more even keel after meals. And, actually there are two types of fiber, one that promotes regularity, and another type that has some special health benefits. The fiber known as "roughage," which helps keep us regular, is called "insoluble fiber." The other type is called "soluble fiber" or the newer term, "functional fiber."

Roughage helps speed the flow of wastes through our digestive tracts, and can help keep us "regular." It may also help reduce the risk of colon cancer. It is found in the skins and pulp of fruits, the seeds in berries, the outer covering of whole grains, and in vegetables.

Soluble fiber has many interesting properties. It too helps promote regularity by making waste more bulky, softer, and easier to move through the intestines. It also thickens the digested food in our small intestines, so that absorption of sugars is slowed. It can soak up cholesterol so that it gets eliminated rather than being absorbed. Soluble fiber is found in oats and barley, fruits (especially apples, pears, and oranges), beans and lentils, and in vegetables.

Even though most Americans get more food than they need each day, most of us get way too little fiber. Guidelines suggest that we should consume at least 25 grams of fiber each day. Most of my private practice clients get less than 12 grams of fiber per day. There are a variety of ways people miss out on high-fiber foods. Beyond salads and potatoes, most of us lack variety in vegetables with our on-the-go eating. Many people say their fresh fruit tends to go bad before they remember to eat it, so they stop buying it. Bagels have replaced whole grain cereals for a quick, on-the-run breakfast. And beans and lentils are not even on the radar screen.

Good Source of Fiber

	Soluble Fiber	Total Fiber
Apple, unpeeled	.4	3.0
Pear, unpeeled	.7	4.6
Raspberries, ½ cup	.3	2.6
Prunes, 5	1.1	3.1
Avocado, ½	1.2	3.8
Sweet Potato, ½ cup	.5	1.9
Broccoli, 2 stalks	.2	1.8
Carrots, ½ cup	.4	1.9
Spaghetti Sauce, ½ cup	.6	3.0
Kidney beans, ½ cup	1.0	4.5
All-bran Cereal, 1/3 cup	.7	8.1
Oatmeal, ¾ cup	1.2	2.7

With the DASH diet, getting sufficient fiber in your diet is part of the plan. You don't even have to think about it.

INTRODUCING MORE FIBER INTO YOUR DIET

Many of us have gotten used to consuming a low fiber diet. In order to help your body adjust to higher amounts of fiber (with all those DASH fruits and vegetables), it can be helpful to go slowly. As we age, some people find that high fiber foods cause discomfort, and they experience intestinal bloating or gas. The gradual approach may allow your body to better adjust to fiber. Try to add 1 to 2 extra fruits or vegetables to your daily intake, and then hold at that level for several days. Then increase again. If you find that you are still uncomfortable, you may want to try one of the fiber digesting supplements. There are several brands on the market, including Beano™.

It is very important to increase your intake of fluid when you add more fiber. You must get at least 8 glasses of fluid per day. A high fiber diet without plenty of fluid will still leave you constipated. (If you have any disease that requires fluid restriction, consult with your physician and a registered dietitian before making any changes in your diet, both in terms of the amount of fluid and in the amount of fiber.)

DASHboard

1. A balanced approach to fat, protein, and carbs is important for health and for a healthy weight.
2. Choose unsaturated fats, especially MUFAs and omega-3 PUFAs. Limit SFA.
3. Good sources of MUFAs are olive oil, canola oil, nuts, and avocados.
4. Good sources of omega-3 fatty acids are fish, such as tuna, salmon, sardines, and herring.
5. High-fat animal foods are the primary source of saturated fats, which should be minimized.
6. For lean meats, choose "select" meats with the words "loin" or "round" in their names.
7. Low-fat and nonfat dairy are low in calories and saturated fats.
8. High-fiber foods may help to control hunger, help to lower cholesterol, and reduce the risk for certain types of cancer.

Tracking my Personal DASH Diet Action Plan

Food sources of healthy fats I will choose, include: _____

_____

_____

_____

_____

Lean or low-fat protein foods I will choose include: _____

_____

_____

_____

_____

High-fiber foods I will choose, include: _____

_____

_____

_____

_____

CHAPTER 10

MINERALS THAT HELP
LOWER BLOOD PRESSURE

Doctors have known for many years that moderation of salt intake can help many people lower their blood
pressure. It has been less well known that several other minerals
can help reduce blood pressure when they are *increased* in our
diets. Diets that are rich in calcium, potassium, and magnesium,
in particular, have been shown to lower blood pressure, and the
majority of Americans do not get enough of these minerals.
Fortunately, this plan will assure that you meet your needs, since
foods rich in these minerals are the foundation of the DASH
diet.

A DASH of Salt

Everyone has heard that lowering salt will lower blood pressure.
Recently there has been some controversy about this broad state-

ment. Some people may be more sensitive than others to the effects of salt or sodium. (We talk about salt almost interchangeably with sodium, since it is the major contributor of sodium to our diets.) And there are several other minerals, such as potassium, calcium, and magnesium that play into the blood pressure equation.

The original DASH investigation used a moderate level of sodium—3,200 milligrams per day—well above the current recommendations. With the DASH diet, blood pressure was lowered significantly, even at this moderately high intake of sodium. But the question remained, what if the salt level were lower, would there be further improvements in blood pressure control?

Recent DASH studies have shown that, in fact, the lower the salt intake with the DASH diet, the more the blood pressure declined. So, yes, watching your sodium intake is still a good thing.

Many studies have shown that people around the world who consume more sodium have higher blood pressures. This sensitivity increases with age. Societies where people do not consume any salt have almost no hypertension, and blood pressure does not increase with age. (In general these people also have low weight, low alcohol consumption, and high levels of physical activity.)

Typically, African Americans are quite sensitive to salt, and blacks have higher rates of hypertension than whites and Hispanics in the U.S. In the DASH study that investigated the benefit of lower salt levels, blacks, and especially black women, responded better than whites to salt restriction. As we age, we tend to become more sensitive to salt.

Interestingly, as much as it seems like gospel that we should all try to lower our sodium intake, there are some studies in the U.S. which have shown that a low intake of sodium is associated with shorter life span.

Further, some people may be at risk of developing increased blood pressure if they adopt a diet that is overly restrictive in sodium. This includes people who have a cluster of symptoms known as metabolic syndrome (see Chapter 7).

Beyond Salt—Calcium, Potassium, and Magnesium

Sodium isn't the only mineral that is important in managing blood pressure. Calcium, magnesium, and potassium are all involved in helping to regulate blood pressure. And, their relationship with blood pressure is generally positive. That is, including more of these minerals in your diet helps to lower blood pressure. An important point to remember is that studies have shown that eating foods rich in these nutrients helps to lower blood pressure. However, studies looking at dietary supplements containing these minerals were mostly unsuccessful in producing the same benefits for blood pressure control.

CALCIUM

Calcium has many interesting health benefits beyond strengthening bones. People who include more calcium in their diets tend to have lower blood pressure, weigh less, have less body fat, and have a lower risk for developing type 2 diabetes. The DASH diet encourages at least 2 to 3 servings a day of low-fat or nonfat dairy foods. I generally recommend 3 to 4 daily servings of dairy to get 1,200 milligrams of calcium, which is the RDA for people over fifty.

The news about all the extra health benefits of dairy is really very exciting. How nice to be able to add foods into your diet that have such positive benefits. Over the last thirty years, Americans' consumption of milk has declined dramatically. Many researchers have noted a connection between decreased consumption of milk and increased rates of obesity and hypertension. It is important to choose low-fat or nonfat dairy foods, as consumption increases. The fat in milk is butterfat, which has a very high saturated fat content. Skim (nonfat) milk, reduced-fat or nonfat cheese, and nonfat yogurt are all great additions to your diet. If you find skim milk too "watery" you may find that low-carb nonfat milk is richer tasting, and it has a whiter color than regular skim milk.

If you are lactose intolerant, you can find lactose-free milk or take lactose-digesting enzyme tablets. The lactose in yogurt has already been broken down by the bacteria that turn milk into yogurt, making it a great choice. Most cheese is also very low in lactose, having less than 1 gram per serving. If you must avoid milk, make sure to choose yogurt with vitamin D added, or consider taking a multivitamin. Vitamin D is essential for absorbing calcium, but it is not found in cheese and many yogurts.

There are many vegetables that are good sources of calcium, and many plant-based foods, such as soy milk, that are formulated to be good sources of calcium, so that even a vegan diet can provide plenty of calcium.

POTASSIUM

A large worldwide study (Intersalt) showed that if potassium were high in relation to sodium, blood pressure was lower. Unfortunately, most Americans do not get enough potassium in their diets. One of the benefits of the DASH diet is that it will automatically increase your intake of potassium while minimizing added salt. The DASH diet encourages 4 to 5 servings of fruits and 4 to 5 servings of vegetables each day, many of which are rich sources of potassium.

Potassium allows the body to get rid of extra fluid so that the heart doesn't have to pump too hard, thereby allowing blood pressure to stay low. It is also important for regulating the heartbeat. Good sources of potassium include most fruits and vegetables, especially oranges, bananas, potatoes, and tomatoes, as shown in the table at the end of this chapter. High amounts of dietary potassium can counteract some of the effects of too much dietary sodium.

Some people are on blood pressure medication that can interfere with excreting potassium, and their doctors may recommend limiting potassium intake. Even though there are many health benefits of potassium, do not use the advice given here to override your doctor's recommendation. If you would like to adopt the DASH diet and have been cautioned about too much potassium, be sure to discuss this with your physician.

MAGNESIUM

Magnesium is another important mineral for keeping blood pressure under control. However, most Americans do not get enough magnesium in their diet. Whole grains are great sources of magnesium, as are nuts and some vegetables and fruits. The tables at the end of this chapter will show you which foods are richest in magnesium.

Shaking the Salt Habit

Many people feel that it is difficult to limit sodium, since it is important for flavoring foods. Salt has been very important throughout human history; many ancient villages were situated to be close to salt deposits. In addition to flavoring, salt was important in preserving foods. The ancient Romans paid their soldiers in salt; the Latin word for salt is the root of the English word salary.

We don't have to give up all salt, but we can make significant reductions through some easy substitutions.

1. Choose frozen vegetables instead of canned. No salt is added to frozen vegetables (without sauce).

2. Choose low- or no-added-salt canned vegetables. Currently there is no frozen alternative to canned tomato

products, so most have relatively high amounts of added salt. You can find canned low-salt or no-added-salt versions of most tomato products.

3. Avoid salt products earlier in the day if you are going to have salt-containing tomato products at dinner. For example, if you are having spaghetti with canned tomato sauce at dinner, avoid canned tuna or other salted foods at breakfast and lunch.

4. Limit cured meats, such as bacon, ham, sausage, hot dogs, etc. The salt that is added to these foods is necessary to preserve the meat. So, limit these foods to once a week or less.

5. Limit canned soups. Make your own soups without added salt.

6. Choose lower salt cheeses, such as Swiss or Lorraine. Use smaller amounts of high salt cheeses. Read labels to check the sodium content of various cheeses.

7. Use fresh fruit as a dessert instead of baked goods, such as cookies, to reduce sodium while increasing fruit servings.

8. Try cucumbers covered in a sweet vinegar, such as rice wine vinegar, red wine vinegar, or balsamic vinegar, rather than pickles.

9. Limit olives and capers.

10. Indulge your salt craving with a ½-ounce serving of potato chips instead of a "Grab Bag™" or similar large-sized serving. You will limit your sodium to only 90 milligrams, and limit the weight consequences, since this portion only has 75 calories. (Yes, this is a surprise. You can include some salted snacks without overdoing sodium.)

11. Choose seasoning mixes without salt, such as lemon pepper mix, Italian seasoning mix, or other seasoning flavors.

12. Forget about salting your fries. If you need seasoning, try spice mixes. At restaurants, where you don't have options, you may find that you don't even miss the salt. (And limiting fries is a good thing for reducing calories and added fats.)

13. Reduce salt in canned beans by rinsing them well in water. If you have the time, let them soak in water for 30 minutes to eliminate even more sodium.

14. Dry beans are an even better choice since they do not have added sodium. Or, choose lentils. They are a quicker substitution, since they don't require long overnight soaking like dry beans.

DASH Diet Mineral-Rich Foods

Since we don't eat minerals, we need to meet our dietary requirements from the foods we eat. (And remember, as we pointed out earlier, dietary mineral supplements have not shown the same benefits as consuming foods rich in these minerals.) The following lists show you which foods are rich in the key blood pressure-lowering minerals. You will also see that these foods are the key DASH diet foods.

Calcium-Rich Foods		
Dairy	**Vegetables**	**Beans**
milk	broccoli	soybeans
yogurt	kale	tofu
cottage cheese	bok choi	
cheese		

Potassium-Rich Foods

Vegetables
asparagus
artichoke
bamboo shoots
beets
broccoli
Brussels sprouts
carrots
beans
cauliflower
celery
kale
mushrooms
okra
potatoes
pumpkin
seaweed
spinach
turnip greens
squash (winter)
sweet potato
tomatoes

Fruits
apricots
avocado
banana
cantaloupe
grapefruit
honeydew
kiwifruit
orange
prunes
strawberries
tangerine
dried fruits
apple
apricots
dates
pear
peach

Cereals and Breads
bran cereals
Mueslix
pumpernickel bread

Nuts
almonds
brazil nuts
cashews
chestnuts
filberts
hazelnuts
peanuts
pecans
pumpkin seeds
sunflower seeds
walnuts

Miscellaneous
coffee
molasses
tea
tofu

Magnesium-Rich Foods

Fruits and Vegetables	Whole Grains	Nuts
avocado	amaranth	pumpkin seeds
banana	barley	sunflower seeds
beet greens	buckwheat	sesame seeds
black-eyed peas	bulgur	almonds
casava	granola	cashews
beans and lentils	millet	flax seeds
figs	oats	hazel nuts
okra	brown rice	brazil nuts
potatoes w/skin	wild rice	peanuts
raisins	rye	walnuts
seaweed	triticale	pistachios
spinach	whole wheat	soybeans
Swiss chard	bran	macadamia
wax beans		nuts
		pecans

DASHboard

1. Avoid salt. Limit canned and processed foods. Limit olives, pickles, and capers. Choose low-salt cheeses. Limit cured meats, such as bacon, ham, and sausages.

2. Include lots of foods rich in potassium, calcium, and magnesium. These include fruits, vegetables, whole grains, dairy, and nuts.

Tracking my Personal DASH Diet Action Plan

I will include the following foods in my diet:

Potassium-rich: _____

_____

_____

Magnesium-rich: _____

_____

_____

Calcium-rich:_____

_____

_____

I will limit sodium by avoiding the following: _____

_____

_____

My low-salt alternatives will be:_____

_____

_____

CHAPTER 11

DECIPHERING FOOD LABELS

Nutrition labels were developed to help people make nutritious food choices. Many of the nutrients that are required on food labels can help people reduce their risk of developing or help manage some very common diseases and conditions, such as heart disease, hypertension, diabetes, and obesity. The key nutrients include calories, total fat, saturated fat, trans fats, cholesterol, sodium, total carbohydrates, and protein.

For someone following the DASH diet, the Nutrition Facts panel can help with making good food choices. Choosing lean meat and poultry and low-fat dairy foods is easy when you can easily determine how much fat is in the food and which types are low in saturated fats. You can make low-sodium choices, and look for high fiber foods—all based on the Nutrition Facts.

Specific information must be shown on the Nutrition Facts panel label, as shown here. In the following sections I will go through the panel, step-by-step to explain the components.

Serving Size

First, you want to know how much is in a serving of the food. In this example (plain yogurt) the serving size is 1 cup, which is the amount in the entire container. If there are multiple servings in a container, the Nutrition Facts panel will help you see this. For example, a bag of microwave popcorn might contain 2 or 3 servings. You need to check to be sure what serving size the calories and nutrients are based on.

Plain Yogurt

Nutrition Facts	
Serving Size 1 cup (248 g)	
Servings per container 1	
Amount Per Serving	
Calories 150 Calories from Fat 35	
	% Daily Value*
Total Fat 4 g	6%
Saturated Fat 2.5 g	12%
Trans Fat 0 g	
Cholesterol 20 mg	7%
Sodium 170 mg	7%
Total Carbohydrate 17 g	6%
Dietary Fiber 0 g	
Sugars 17 g	
Protein 13g	
Vitamin A 4% • Vitamin C 6%	
Calcium 40% • Iron 0%	
*Percent Daily Values are based on a 2,000 calorie diet.	

In general, for multi-serving packages, there are standardized serving sizes. However, it gets a little confusing to compare single-serving containers of different sizes. For example, the standard serving of potato chips is 1 ounce. However, if you have a ½-ounce bag of chips, that is a serving, for that package. For a 1½-ounce bag, the serving size for that package is the entire 1½ ounces, since it is assumed that you will consume the entire bag.

Cereals are one of the most challenging foods to judge a serving size. The standard serving size is 1 ounce. Serving size by volume can range from ¼ cup to 1¼ cups. And with some very dense cereals, such as Grape Nuts™, the label serving size is ½ cup, which is 2 ounces, or 2 DASH diet servings. It is very important to check the serving size and see how that compares with the serving size you want for your calorie needs in the DASH diet.

Total Calories and Calories From Fat

Total calories are related to serving size. The calories from fat give you an idea of the nutrient density. Foods that are high in calories and without significant vitamins, minerals, or protein, are considered to have a low nutrient density. They bring calories, but not much nutritional value. If someone eats a high-fat diet, it is possible that he or she could be getting adequate calories, but still be malnourished. If you consume too much high-fat foods, you may go over your target calories even without eating much food. So, go easy on foods that have more than 30% of their calories from fat.

Nutrient Composition

The next section of the food label shows the grams of various nutrients in a serving, and the percent daily values. The daily values percentage can often be very confusing. Many people look at the percentage and think it represents the percent of the nutrient in the food. Using the yogurt example, the 4 grams of fat represent 6% of the requirement for a day, based on a 2,000-calorie diet. It doesn't mean that 6% of the calories in the yogurt come from fat. In fact, since 35 of the 150 calories come from fat (from the top section), 23% of the calories are from fat. It is important for controlling cholesterol to choose foods that are low in saturated and trans fats.

Sodium and occasionally potassium are listed in this section. You, obviously, want to limit sodium and choose foods that are rich in potassium.

In the carbohydrate section you will find total carbohydrates, fiber, and sugars. The carbohydrate that isn't sugar or fiber is mostly starch, which you can compute by subtracting fiber and sugar from the total carbohydrate value. Fiber content may also be segmented further to show grams of soluble fiber.

Additional vitamins and minerals with special health concerns are shown in the bottom section of the Nutrition Facts panel. Vitamin C, Vitamin A, calcium, and iron content must be included on the label. Manufacturers may also list additional vitamins and minerals, if they choose.

Ingredients

Another requirement for food labels is that they must include an ingredient list. If you are concerned about cholesterol, you may want to go easy on foods that contain hydrogenated or partially hydrogenated fats.

The ingredient list is another way to check how much sugar has been added to a food. Some of the many terms that indicate sugar include high fructose corn syrup, grape juice (and other fruit juices), corn syrup, honey, molasses, dextrose, fructose, and lactose.

Since ingredients must be listed in order by weight (from the highest to the lowest), having many sources of sugar can help the manufacturer disguise the importance of sugar in the overall product formula. The Nutrition Facts panel will provide better information on the amount of sugar in a specific food. Many healthy DASH diet foods naturally contain sugars (such as fruits, yogurt, and milk) and should not be avoided, unless they contain lots of extra added-sugars. Again, read the ingredient list to see if sugars have been added, and compare calories for comparable foods.

DASHboard

1. Food labels help you limit intake of sodium, and saturated and trans fats.

2. Read food labels closely to check serving sizes.

3. Use food labels to limit calories.

4. Use food labels to find foods rich in potassium and calcium.

Tracking my Personal DASH Diet Action Plan

I will read food labels to choose healthy DASH diet foods:

❏ Never

❏ Rarely

❏ Often

❏ I already read food labels

CHAPTER 12

VEGETABLES FOR PICKY EATERS

This chapter reveals the "true confessions" of a picky eater and former vegetable-hater. As a child, the only cooked vegetables I ate were sweet corn (really a grain and not a vegetable) and potatoes. Sometimes I would eat green beans or wax beans, but not often. I did like many raw vegetables, such as tomatoes, lettuce, carrots, and celery. But I would reject any of these foods if they were cooked.

Now I am a fairly adventurous eater. What changed? First, I got older. Children taste foods more intensely than adults. As we become older, we may find that foods we didn't like as children aren't quite so bad anymore. And we may find that we actually *like* some of these previously "distasteful" foods. Check out your adult taste buds by trying some new vegetables.

Another factor in our changing preferences is that we have changed how we cook vegetables. It is trendy to cook vegetables just until "crisp-tender" rather than boiling them until they are quite soft. Cooking vegetables for a shorter time keeps the flavor milder and sweeter. Gentle microwaving and steaming are less likely to form the strong flavors that we associate with some vegetables, such as members of the cabbage family including broccoli and cauliflower, and help avoid mushy textures.

Many things contribute to an appreciation of vegetables. The following ideas have worked for me and for my patients. There will probably still be vegetables that you really can't "stomach," so don't feel like a failure if you are resistant to some. The goal is just to expand your comfort zone. Several of the following suggestions are sure to click with you as you expand your palate.

Grow Your Meal

A fun way to get more vegetables into your life is to plant some vegetables in your garden. Fresh foods taste better, and it is very satisfying to create something of value by growing your own food. There are many types of vegetables you can grow, even if you only have a small space. Try one or two, or several, for a real harvest bounty.

Peppers come in many colors and add adventure to your garden. Bell peppers in red, yellow, orange, ivory, and purple add as much color as flowering plants. The hotter peppers, like red jalapeños and orange habañeros, are a great way to spice up your plantings. Peppers are excellent sources of nutrients and antioxidants, such as carotenoids (orange, yellow, and red colors) and vitamin C. The cool crunch adds extra texture to your salads and makes a colorful addition to an appetizer tray. Jalapeños add zest to fresh salsa made with tomatoes or fruit. You may get added health benefits from the capsaicin, which puts heat into hot peppers.

Red cabbage looks like a big lush flower in your garden. It makes a great accent between your plants, and on the table. It adds color to salads and can be braised for a succulent side dish. Broccoli is a fast grower and can quickly produce a tender, mild vegetable for your dinner plate. Both red cabbage and broccoli are members of the cruciferous vegetable family, and are rich sources of vitamin C, beta carotene, and other substances that may help protect against cancer. When you pick them straight from the garden and eat them right away, there is less chance for losing storage-sensitive nutrients, such as vitamin C.

Tomatoes are a perennial garden favorite, and produce fruit with much more flavor than store-bought ones. New varieties, such as grape tomatoes, produce lavish harvests and are incredibly sweet. They add color and great flavor to salads or can be simmered in sauces for entrées. Tomatoes are rich in carotenoids, especially lycopene, a powerful antioxidant. Yellow tomatoes don't contain lycopene, but make colorful additions to dinners and brighten up your garden. Tomatoes are a great source of vitamin C.

You can sneak onions in between your flowers and vegetables, where they may protect your plants from insects. And, they can also protect you. The allium found in foods in the onion family may reduce the risk for several types of cancer. Other easy-to-grow choices from the onion family include chives, leeks, shallots, and garlic. They add flavor to many types of foods to increase your dining pleasure, and they are good for you. Garlic has been shown to help reduce cholesterol, while it adds nuances to sauces and salads.

Climbing vegetables can grow up a fence or a wall or a balcony rail. Green beans, wax beans, peas, and cucumbers add greenery to your yard, without taking up space. (And they stay cleaner when they are off the ground.) Fresh baby green beans or the skinny French *haricots verts* have a tenderness and sweetness you miss in the varieties found in the grocery store. Low in calories and good sources of vitamin C, beans are terrific additions to summertime dinners. A wall of lettuce can be fun if you are handy. The lettuces grow in a bag filled with soilless growing medium, and peek out from the branches of a lattice. You won't need trips to the grocery store for fresh greenery. Darker colored lettuce can be a good source of carotenoids, vitamins E and K, as well as potassium.

If you have lots of space, you can add yellow crookneck squash and zucchini. Low calorie members of the squash family, they are terrific sliced in a salad or sautéed as a side dish. They can also be cut in chunks to be skewered for a shish kabob. The starchier winter squashes will last further into the fall, and with their yellow-orange color, they are obviously very rich in carotenoids, especially beta carotene. Roasted at a high temperature in the oven, their sweetness will complement a winter dinner.

Beans, Beans, Beans

Most Americans are reluctant to add beans to their diet. (Here we are referring to legumes such as soybeans, kidney beans, lentils, and navy beans. Green beans don't count in this category, since they are primarily the bean pods.) Legumes are rich in vegetable protein and soluble fiber, which lowers cholesterol.

Some people don't know what to do with beans, some people don't like the flavor, and some people have texture aversions to beans. There are tricks to get around any of these concerns. If you don't like the texture or flavor of soy, there are some great soy-based meat substitutes available at your supermarket to make it easy for you to add the health benefits of soy to your diet. You may already be familiar with soy-based vegetarian burgers.

Did you know that there are many other soy-based products, such as "chicken" nuggets, Buffalo wings, hot dogs, and even ground "meat?" These fit the bill for fast, easy meals that include all the advantages of soy, such as lowering cholesterol, improving the absorption of calcium, adding beneficial fiber, and providing phytochemicals which may help lower the risk of some kinds of cancer.

Women may be looking for ways to incorporate soy into their diets for many health reasons, including relieving some symptoms of menopause. Chocolate-based soy "milk" drinks provide another tasty way to add the benefits of soy to your diet.

I admit to not liking the unenhanced taste of soy. I spent several years working as a food scientist at a soy company, and I can detect the soy flavor in any food . . . or so I thought. As a food science instructor, I found I needed to add more vegetarian recipes to my courses to accommodate vegetarian students. I discovered that the new tofu recipes do taste great, and they do not taste like soy. Soy tends to mask the flavor of other foods, making them taste bland. Adding extra seasonings and spices, or marinades, will ensure a full-flavored dish.

In addition to my soy aversion, I will admit that I didn't like the texture of beans. But I have now learned to enjoy them. A bean-rich chili can be an easy way to introduce beans into your diet. The chili can also include meat, to enhance its familiarity. I add lots of frozen vegetables, everything from corn and red peppers, blends of cauliflower, broccoli, and carrots, to frozen diced green peppers and onions (recipe in Chapter 14). After cooking, everything tastes like chili. With all the different textures, you won't notice the beans. Be creative and find your own vegetable mixtures to include.

Go on a culinary adventure. Beans are an important part of the Mediterranean diet. Many finer Italian restaurants have at least one bean dish on the menu. They know how to prepare beans to make them flavorful. The seasonings, sauce, pasta, and beans all complement each other for a fabulous dining experience. In my food classes, I have added Italian pasta and bean dishes that even the "bean-averse" discover to be very tasty. Latin American and Caribbean dishes are often based on beans, and can provide additional new food items.

The cuisine of India is largely vegetarian. At an Indian restaurant, instead of choosing Americanized meat or chicken dishes, try some vegetarian choices, with beans providing the protein.

Try Middle Eastern falafel or hummus dip; both are made from chickpeas (garbanzo beans). The Chinese were the first to domesticate soy more than 4,000 years ago. Soy is an important part of many traditional Chinese foods, and the cuisine of its neighbor, Japan. Choose traditional foods at these restaurants, rather than the Americanized dishes.

You may enjoy boxed meal mixes (containing pasta, beans, and seasonings), such as Bean Cuisine®, that come with quick-cooking beans. Every client to whom I have recommended these products really loves them. Even vegetable-hating clients find that the bean dishes taste great, and are an easy way to introduce beans into their meals. On the back of the box are recommendations for adding other vegetables and some kind of liquid, such as vegetable or chicken broth. You could add meat or chicken to make the dishes more familiar. These meals are ready to eat in 15 minutes, and only take one pot to prepare.

The "bean squeamish" can try a few bites of the beans, and still have lots of "regular" food to eat if they really don't like the beans.

Cater to the Inner Child—Sneaking in Vegetables

Many children find that vegetables, especially cooked ones, taste too strong. Fortunately, as we get older, we don't taste our foods as intensely as children do. Since I counsel children, as well as adults, I have learned ways to sneak vegetables into other dishes, and to recycle ideas from childhood vegetable favorites.

Some mothers become experts in tricking their kids into eating their vegetables. Maybe you can trick yourself. Why not purée some vegetables and add them to your spaghetti sauce? If you are bean-averse, you could even purée some beans. Some moms add them to hamburger or meatloaf. Sloppy Joes are everyone's childhood favorite. Add several handfuls of frozen onions and green peppers to the meat while it is browning. In my stir-fry dishes I add fistfuls of broccoli slaw, which become sweet when stir-fried and look like noodles. Carrot cake and zucchini bread are good sources of vegetables (albeit higher calorie), and they taste great.

Remember the salads your mother used to make when you were a kid (if you grew up in the fifties)? Rediscover the fun. How about diced vegetables floating in a gelatin mold? Carrots and raisin salad. Cole slaw with pineapple. The ever-popular three-bean salad. Tomatoes stuffed with tuna salad. And yes, tuna and chicken salad can provide another way to hide some vegetables. We all add diced celery. How about adding some finely diced red peppers, shredded carrots, or cucumbers?

And while we are on the subject of fifties vegetables, the infamous green bean casserole is still a perennial favorite for Thanksgiving.

Soups are another childhood favorite that entice us to try some vegetables. Tomato soup was always my special comfort food.

How about vegetable soup with or without chicken or beef? Split pea soup is a way to sneak in some legumes rich in soluble fiber. Cabbage soup is a special sweet treat. While we would like to limit cream soups, there are many types that include vegetables, and occasionally can provide some added variety to your vegetable repertoire.

Don't forget vegetable broth, which can be added to many dishes. While the broth lacks the fiber of whole vegetables, it still adds phytochemicals and other vegetable nutrients. Homemade soups help keep sodium under control.

Who Says Carrots Don't Belong on a Sandwich?

I love salad bars in grocery stores. They are a great place to find cut-up fresh vegetables. Expand your ideas of what can go on a sandwich by experimenting with salad toppings. Tomatoes and lettuce on your sandwich are a cliché.

Break out of the rut! Grated carrots, slawed red cabbage, and sliced radishes make great toppings. Don't forget some sliced green, red, and yellow bell peppers. Add some fresh sliced Bermuda onion for tang, or sprouts for extra crunch. Try broccoli slaw. Baby spinach or mesclun add an adult flavor to the lowly sandwich. Sliced black or green olives are special treats (and full of healthy monounsaturated fat).

How to Avoid Ruining the Vegetables

We all remember George Bush (the first President Bush) saying that he didn't like broccoli and didn't want it served to him anymore. (Although why it took him until he was one year into his presidency to work up the courage to make his wishes known, is a completely different issue.)

Broccoli and other foods in the cabbage family can develop strong sulfur odors if they are over-cooked. Green beans become mushy and lose their bright green color when cooked too long. (Although there are regional and cultural differences in the degree of tenderness people prefer.)

The new cuisine encourages gently cooking vegetables. This preserves more of the heat-sensitive nutrients and the natural sweetness of fresh produce.

To have milder tasting broccoli, and other foods in the cruciferous vegetable family, such as cabbage, cauliflower, and kale, choose the freshest produce. During the summer, grow your own, or go to the farmer's market to get really fresh vegetables. Older vegetables will develop more of the strong sulfur odor on cooking.

If you are cooking them by boiling in water, leave the lid off. That allows the volatile sulfur compounds to evaporate into the air, instead of being trapped in the cooking water. Cook small portions in the microwave. The shorter cooking times won't cause strong flavors to develop. Steaming is another terrific way to avoid off-flavors.

Don't add baking soda to your vegetables. Although baking soda helps preserve the bright green color of many vegetables, it makes vegetables very soft and mushy, which is a turn-off to many picky eaters.

Don't add acid too early when cooking your beans. If you are cooking beans to be used in baked beans or the barbecued lentils featured in our recipe section, don't add tomato products too early in the cooking process. The acid will make the beans more difficult to cook and tenderize, and the overly chewy texture is sure to repel the newly reformed vegetable-hater.

On The Cutting Edge and Raw

Raw fresh vegetables have the mildest and sweetest flavor. Either go to the salad bar or sharpen up your knives. School lunch programs take advantage of the fact that kids will eat their carrots if they are given some ranch dressing for dipping. Any salad dressing livens up raw broccoli, carrots, celery, or cucumbers. Radishes, peppers, jicama all compete to make a crisp, cool crunch.

Dips made with nonfat sour cream remake vegetables into party favorites. My favorite is medium-hot salsa mixed into nonfat sour cream. You can alter any of your dip recipes to make them into healthy additions to your appetizer platters.

Why not try some bean dip or one of the fruit-based salsas to break the monotony of vegetables with spinach dip? (Although we are not casting aspersions on this classic dip.)

You can make a salad of raw vegetables that don't fall into the ordinary category. Try zucchini, yellow squash, cucumbers, or beets. You can blanch (lightly cook) a variety of colorful vegetables, such as yellow and red peppers, broccoli, and thinly sliced carrots with some cauliflower, then quick-chill and top with dressing for a still crunchy, new kind of salad.

Sweeten Up the Pot

There are several easy chef-inspired tricks for sweetening vegetables. Onions get sweet when they are "sweated," which means they are cooked slowly over a low heat to caramelize the natural sugars. Try an onion confit. Zucchini and summer squash become delightfully sweet and flavorful when sautéed over medium heat in a tiny bit of olive oil. And jicama makes a surprisingly sweet treat when sautéed.

Roasting is another way to caramelize the sugars and bring out hidden richness in vegetables. Try roasting winter squash, such as acorn or butternut, at higher temperatures (450°) to enhance sweetness. You will find that you don't need to top with added sugar to get rich flavor. Bell peppers roasted over an open flame or heated in the oven, quickly yield their skin when wrapped in a bag for several minutes after roasting. Slice into strips, which are absolutely heavenly. You can also purée the roasted peppers for a sauce. Maybe you won't notice that you are eating vegetables and that it just happens to be good for you.

Other vegetables where the flavors become fabulous when cooked at elevated temperatures include onions, carrots, parsnips, tomatoes, oh—and best of all—sweet potatoes. It is hard to imagine that you could make them sweeter, but try roasting sweet potatoes at 450° for one hour. You won't need any topping and not a bit of butter. For even more suggestions on everything from broccoli to beets to artichokes, I recommend Barbara Kafka's *Roasting* (Morrow, 1995).

Salad Days

Many people find that raw vegetables are more palatable. Salads make a great vehicle for a variety of vegetables. So expand your interests beyond green stuff. Check out the sidebar to get unstuck from your normal routine. When you choose greens, mix it up. Remember, darker green leaves will have more nutrients. Think about choosing romaine, spinach, watercress, red or green leaf lettuce, endive, bib, or escarole. Frizzé or mache are interesting French variations for your salads. Expand your color choices by adding radicchio, mesclun, or red cabbage.

Again, salad bars are great for quick healthy meals. You only buy food that you actually eat. There's no waste! When you buy head lettuce you may end up throwing out half its weight due to brown or rotting leaves. Why bother? Someone else can throw away the unusable parts, and you can pick the best leaves.

Tops for Your Salad

romaine	iceberg	mesclun
watercress	red leaf	endive
bib	loose leaf	escarole
radicchio	mache	frizzé
hot peppers	olives	cucumbers
radishes	sprouts	zucchini
yellow squash	tomatoes	onions
spinach	celery	grated carrots
red cabbage	broccoli slaw	kidney beans
green beans		

bell peppers: red, yellow, orange, ivory, purple, and green

At the salad bar, you can also choose salad toppings to add a variety of vegetables, without filling your refrigerator with rotting, partially used fresh vegetables. Buy what you need for one or two days. And get extra to use on your sandwiches.

If it's a really great salad bar, they will also have cut up fruit to make it easy to add fruits to your day. Choose some cantaloupe, pineapple, watermelon, or strawberries. You can see what they look like without skin, and only pick the most flavorful, freshest pieces. And again, you can choose plenty of variety without any waste.

DASHboard

1. Many people don't like vegetables. They need some tricks to add more veggies into their diet.
2. Grow your own. Fresh vegetables are always best.
3. Beans can add variety to your meals.
4. Sneak in the veggies.
5. Top your sandwich with cut-up veggies.
6. Avoid overcooking vegetables to keep the flavor milder.
7. Raw veggies may be more appealing to people who don't like most vegetables.
8. Salad bars are great sources for cut-up raw veggies. Top your salad with a variety of colorful vegetables.

Tracking my Personal DASH Diet Action Plan

Three vegetables I will include in my diet this week:_____

_____

_____

_____

One bean dish I will try: _____

_____

Two new salad toppers I will try: _____

_____

_____

CHAPTER 13

SUPER-FAST DASH DINING

You have made the commitment to the DASH diet. Some nights you think you just don't have the time to prepare a healthy dinner. How can you make it super quick and easy? Following is a system that is boiled down to the simplest structure.

Super-Simple DASH

Let's make it very simple to track your calorie level and balance the DASH diet servings for your calorie needs. At the end of this chapter is another type of check off form which may be helpful for planning meals. It contains a suggested distribution of food groups for meals and snacks for several calorie levels. You can download larger copies of this form at http://dashdiet.org/forms.asp.

Following is a simplified outline of meals for these calorie levels (based on the form) to help you with your planning.

1,200-Calorie Meals

Breakfast
Whole grain cereal
Whole wheat toast
Nonfat milk
Juice
Fruit for the cereal

Lunch
Half sandwich with whole grain bread, 2 oz. meat, light cheese, topped with veggies
Milk

Snack
Fruit
Nuts

Dinner
3 oz. Meat
Salad with dressing
Vegetables
Small dessert

1,600-Calorie Meals

Breakfast
Whole grain cereal
Whole wheat toast with jam or margarine
Nonfat milk
Juice
Fruit for the cereal

Snack
Light cheese and crackers

Lunch
Sandwich with whole grain bread, 2 oz. meat, light cheese
Salad with dressing
Yogurt

Snack
Fruit
Nuts

Dinner
3 oz. Meat
Rice or Pasta
Salad with dressing
Vegetables
Bread
Fruit
Small dessert

2,000-Calorie Meals

Breakfast
Whole grain cereal
2 slices whole wheat toast with jam or margarine
Nonfat milk
Juice
Fruit for the cereal

Snack
Light cheese and crackers

Lunch
Sandwich with whole grain bread, 3 oz. meat, light cheese
Salad with dressing
Cookies
Yogurt

Snack
Fruit
Nuts

Dinner

4 oz. Meat
Rice or Pasta
Salad with dressing
Vegetables
Bread
Fruit
Small dessert

Super-Fast, Last-Minute Meals

Breakfast, lunches, and snacks are relatively easy to pull together fast. However, many people struggle with dinner. You need super-simple dinner meals. Use the check off list to see what you still need at dinnertime to complete your DASH diet plan for the entire day. Then use these ultra-simple meal ideas.

Start with chicken or pork chops, fresh or frozen. There is no need to thaw the frozen chicken or pork.

Cook in a 375°-400° oven for 45 minutes if frozen, 35-40 minutes for fresh. You can use any kind of oven-safe pan; I often use a glass pie pan. You can add a variety of toppings to make the meals interesting. The meat should be nicely browned when done.

Choose one of the following toppings to make it tasty:

- ♥ 2 T BBQ sauce during last 5 minutes of cooking.
- ♥ 2 T Italian dressing.
- ♥ Salt free seasonings: lemon pepper, Italian seasoning mix, etc.
- ♥ 1 pat of margarine on top of chicken at beginning of cooking process, plus some seasonings.

Shaded boxes indicate desirable extra servings of low fat or nonfat dairy and non-starchy vegetables.

Circled grain boxes indicate minimum servings of whole grains.

Fruit serving size is 4 oz. for 1200 - 1600 calories, and 6 oz. for 2000 - 2400 calories.

For weight control, choose non-starchy vegetables for servings in excess of 5 per day. (Starchy vegetables include potatoes and winter squash.)

If you have more than 3 dairy per day (which is a good idea), remove 1 oz. meat for each extra dairy serving.

Key: G = grain, F = fruit, V = vegetable, D = dairy, M = meat, fish, poultry, egg, N= nuts or beans, O = fats, sugars				
	1200 calories	1600 calories	2000 calories	2400 calories
Breakfast	1 - 2 G 1 - 2 F 1 D	1 - 2 G 1 - 2 F 1 D 1 O	2 - 3 G 2 F 1 D 1 O	2 - 3 G 2 F 1 D 1 O
Lunch	1 - 2 G 1 - 2 V 1 - 2 D 2 oz M 1 O	1 - 3 G 1 F 1 - 2 V 1 - 2 D 2 oz M 1 O	2 - 3 G 1 F 2 V 1 - 2 D 3 oz M 1 O	2 - 3 G 1 F 2+ V 1 - 2 D 4 oz M 2 O
Snacks	0 - 1 F 0 - 1 D 0 - 1 N	0 - 1 G 0 - 1 F 0 - 1 D 0 - 1 N	0 - 1 G 0 - 1 F 0 - 1 D 0 - 1 N	1 - 2 G 0 - 1 F 1 D 0 - 1 N
Dinner	0 - 1 G 2 - 3 V 3 oz M 1 O	2 - 3 G 1 F 2 - 3 V 3 oz M 1 O	2 - 3 G 1 F 2 - 3 V 4 oz M 1 O	5 oz M 1 F 2 - 3+ V 3 - 4 G 2 O
Daily Totals G F V D M N O	▢▢▢ ▢▢▢▢ ▢▢▢▢■ ▢▢▢ ▢▢▢▢▢ ▢ ▢▢	▢▢▢▢▢▢ ▢▢▢▢▢ ▢▢▢▢▢■ ▢▢▢■ ▢▢▢▢▢ ▢ ▢▢▢	▢▢▢▢▢▢▢▢▢ ▢▢▢▢▢ ▢▢▢▢▢■ ▢▢▢■ ▢▢▢▢▢▢▢ ▢ ▢▢▢▢	▢▢▢▢▢▢▢▢▢▢▢ ▢▢▢▢▢ ▢▢▢▢▢▢■■ ▢▢▢■ ▢▢▢▢▢▢▢▢▢ ▢ ▢▢▢▢▢

✓ Shaded boxes indicate desirable extra servings of low fat or nonfat dairy and non-starchy vegetables.
✓ Circled grain boxes indicate minimum servings of whole grains.
✓ Fruit serving size is 4 oz for 1200 - 1600 calories, and 6 oz for 2000 - 2400 calories.
✓ For weight control, choose non-starchy vegetables for servings in excess of 5 per day. (Starchy vegetables include potatoes and winter squash.)
✓ If you have more than 3 dairy per day (which is a good idea), remove 1 oz meat for each extra dairy serving.

Pair any of these dishes with a quick salad, either from the salad bar or from bagged salad mixes, and some microwaved frozen vegetables. This is super fast, easy to pull together, and while the meal is cooking, you have time to decompress from the day (or better yet, get some exercise). Step-by-step photos are on the Website at http://dashdiet.org/superfast.asp.

Another tip for making super-fast healthy dinners is to make larger portions on the weekends (for example, using the recipes for Pile It On! Chili, Sloppy Joes, meaty spaghetti sauce, or any of the bean recipes), and then reheat for a quick weeknight meal. Or warm up restaurant leftovers. For either of these main dish solutions, add a salad and frozen vegetables and you are on track for the DASH diet.

DASHboard

1. Track your DASH diet servings for your calorie needs on the form in this chapter.
2. Make super-fast meals that free up time to relax or exercise.
3. Use weekends to make large portions of key recipes that are rich in vegetables and beans to reheat on week night.

Tracking my Personal DASH Diet Action Plan

Three super-fast dinners I can prepare include: _____

_____

_____

_____

_____

_____

_____

CHAPTER 14

DASH TRACKS, KEEPING TRACK

How do you know if you are really getting on track with the DASH Diet Action Plan? Behavior change is more likely to be successful if you monitor your progress. All through this book you have indicated specific changes you plan to make to adopt the DASH Diet Action Plan and control your blood pressure. It is helpful to track your food intake, exercise, and weight to see how your actions pay off in terms of lowering your blood pressure. Larger copies of all of these forms are available on our Website at http://dashdiet.org/forms.asp. You can download them as many times as you want, to continue to track your progress.

In this book we have two different types of forms for tracking your food intake. They are found in Chapter 2 and Chapter 13.

Blood Pressure Log		
Blood pressure readings	Systolic (top reading)	Diastolic (bottom reading)
Before starting DASH Diet		
Day 1		
Day 2		
Day 3		
Day 4		
Day 5		
Day 6		
Day 7		
Day 8		
Day 9		
Day 10		
Day 11		
Day 12		
Day 13		
Day 14		
Day 15		
Day 16		
Day 17		
Day 18		
Day 19		
Day 20		
Day 21		

Choose the form that seems most useful for you. In this chapter we add forms to track exercise, weight, blood pressure, and overall health and well-being.

The blood pressure log allows you to track how you are responding to the DASH diet. On the first line, write in your typical blood pressure readings before starting the DASH diet. Hopefully, your blood pressure will improve as you change your eating style, lose weight, and add exercise. As a reminder, if your blood pressure is 140/90, 140 is the systolic reading and 90 is the diastolic reading.

Use the exercise log to monitor the activity you perform. Remember, set a goal of doing something active every day. If you can't do 30 or more minutes at one time, schedule three or more 10-minute sessions.

Exercise Log			
Day	Type of Activity	Time	How do I feel?
1			
2			
3			
4			
5			
6			
7			

Getting to a healthier weight or maintaining a healthy weight is important for controlling blood pressure. The following form will provide a convenient way to keep track of your progress with weight control.

Weight Log	
Goal weight	
Initial weight	
Week 1	
Week 2	
Week 3	
Week 4	
Week 5	
Week 6	
Week 7	
Week 8	

Additional benefits of making changes in diet, weight, and activity are improved mood, higher energy level, and enhanced sense of control over your health. A diary of your feelings may provide you with additional information that will help you sustain your behavior changes. On the following page is a model for a simple diary to track how the DASH Diet Action Plan is affecting your life.

And, all of these forms are available for downloading in larger format at http://dashdiet.org/forms.asp.

Overall DASH Diet Outcome Log	
	Mood, energy level, self-confidence, etc.
Initial	
Week 1	
Week 2	
Week 3	
Week 4	
Month 2	
Month 3	
Month 4	
Month 5	
Month 6	

DASHboard

1. Track your progress.
2. Track eating.
3. Track exercise.
4. Track weight.
5. Track blood pressure.
6. Track your new attitude.

Tracking my Personal DASH Diet Action Plan

Forms I will use to track my DASH Diet Action Plan progress:
- ❏ DASH Diet Meal Check Off
- ❏ DASH Diet Calorie Check Off
- ❏ Blood Pressure Log
- ❏ Exercise Log
- ❏ Weight Log
- ❏ Overall DASH Diet Outcome Log

CHAPTER 15

THE DASH
KITCHEN MAKEOVER

The key to making the DASH diet work for you is to set the stage for success—and the kitchen is your stage for eating. In this chapter I will help you design a set for healthy eating, the DASH diet way.

The key DASH diet foods are fruits, vegetables, low-fat and nonfat dairy, nuts and beans, lean meats, fish, and poultry. Keeping these foods on hand will make it easy to follow the DASH diet. If, on the other hand, you keep lots of candy, chips, cookies, and ice cream in your home, you will be inclined to fill up on the wrong foods. The foods you keep on hand will determine what you eat. Keeping lots of the right foods on hand will make it easy to grab foods or make a last-minute meal that will keep you on track with the DASH diet.

Let's take it step by step.

Stock Up

You will want to stock your cupboards and refrigerator with staples that allow you to make a variety of meals without having to run to the store every day (unless, of course, you like to grocery shop daily). The lists that follow will provide a foundation for making it easy to DASH every day.

Making Great DASH Choices

It is easy to make great choices by buying whole grains, fruits, and vegetables. But what about dairy and meats, fish, and poultry?

The key to a heart-healthy diet is choosing foods that are low in saturated fats. In the dairy group, a great choice is nonfat (skim) milk. It has all the calcium, protein, and none of the saturated fats that are found in whole milk and most other dairy foods. If you are lactose intolerant, you can find lactose-free milk or take lactose-digesting enzymes to ease digestion. Another option is low-carb milk (technically a dairy beverage, not milk), which has the added benefit of extra calcium, extra protein, and an extra rich taste compared with regular nonfat milk.

Nonfat yogurt is equally good. If you are watching calories, choose yogurts with little or no added sugars. The labels on yogurt can be confusing as to sugar content because of the milk sugar. (And for carb counters, most of the milk sugar has been converted to lactic acid in yogurts, although the label does not reflect this.) Choose yogurts with less than 120 calories for 6- to 8 ounce servings. As an added benefit, most people with lactose intolerance can handle yogurt very well.

When choosing cheese, buy reduced-fat or nonfat cheese for home. When you are dining out, you generally don't have a low-fat cheese option available, so have it when you can. Make sure your home is stocked with reduced-fat cheese. Cheeses are very low in lactose.

Which is better, butter or margarine? A soft margarine that doesn't contain trans fats is your best choice. For special baking or cooking, you can occasionally use butter, as long as you use it rarely. I choose butter for special meals for its flavor, but I rarely use either margarine or butter as part of my routine diet.

Meats and poultry are other common sources of saturated fats. In general, choosing select grades of beef, and cuts with the words "round" or "loin" in their names will give you lean cuts. Appendix A provides you with a list of beef, pork, and poultry cuts and their calorie and fat contents. And of course, skinless chicken and turkey are low in saturated fat.

Most fish and seafood is very low in saturated fat. While shrimp may be high in cholesterol, it is still considered to be a good choice as part of a heart-healthy diet since it is very low in fat. (As long as it is not fried or swimming in butter.) Most fatty fish contain the omega-3 fatty acids that are considered to be very heart healthy. Even fatty fish are still in the lean range when compared with meat and poultry.

Coconut oil is a surprising source of saturated fat. This may be found in popcorn, especially commercially prepared fresh popcorn.

Trans fats are found in many baked goods, such as pastries, snack crackers, and pie crusts. The food labels now list trans fat content so that you can choose to limit these foods. You can limit trans fats by avoiding foods with hydrogenated or partially hydrogenated fats.

Staples

Canned/Bottled/Dry
diced tomatoes, no added salt
tomato sauce, no added salt
tomato paste, no added salt
kidney beans, no added salt
black beans, no added salt
lentils
tuna, canned in water,
    low-salt
canned salmon, low-salt
canned chicken, low-salt
extra virgin olive oil
canola oil
vegetable oil
white and/or yellow corn meal
oatmeal
cereals without added sugar,
    and high in fiber
various types of pasta: rotini,
    spaghetti, angel hair, shells,
    linguine, etc.
nuts, unsalted

Spices and Herbs
bag of onions
bulbs of garlic
shallots
dry spices including basil,
    oregano, parsley flakes,
    thyme, marjoram, paprika,
    rosemary, ginger, poultry
    seasoning, sage, onion
    powder, garlic powder, etc.
taco sauce or seasonings
chili mix
salt substitutes, including
    lemon-pepper

reduced-sodium soy sauce
stir-fry sauces/mixes,
    low-sodium
potato seasoning mixes
Worcestershire sauce

Frozen
individual and mixed
    vegetables
sliced pepper and onion mix
diced onions
diced green peppers
frozen skinless boneless
    chicken breasts
frozen 95% lean ground
    sirloin (& patties)
pizza crusts
corn or flour tortillas
whole wheat pitas
frozen yogurt, with no
    added sugar
frozen fruit

Refrigerated
lemon juice
lime juice
dark green lettuces
baby carrots
grape tomatoes
grated carrots
sliced carrots
coleslaw mix
broccoli slaw
salad dressings
sliced deli meats, low-sodium
barbecue sauce, low-sodium
whole wheat bread
oatmeal bran bread
ketchup, low-salt
mustard

Fresh From the Market

Fresh Additions
salad bar for fresh, cut-up
   items:
lettuce
radishes
peppers
onions
carrots
broccoli
cauliflower
red cabbage
cucumber
beets
fresh fruit

Produce Counter
fresh fruits, vegetables, greens,
   fresh herbs

Meat Counter
fresh fish
lean meat, poultry
(see Appendix A)

Dairy
Low-fat or nonfat, low-
   sodium cheeses: cheddar,
   Swiss, Colby/jack,
   Parmesan, Romano, moz-
   zarella, sliced and grated
   cheeses
light individually packaged
   cheeses such as Baby Bel™,
   Laughing Cow™, string
   cheese, Kraft 2% Singles™,
   2% or 1% cottage cheese
nonfat yogurt, artificially
   sweetened
skim milk or low-carb skim
   milk
egg substitutes
eggs or omega-3-rich eggs

Equipment

Having the right equipment will make your life easier, whether you like to cook or don't want to spend your time cooking.

- ♥ Countertop grill. This allows the quick preparation of lean meats, fish, and poultry. The newer versions have removable grill surfaces for easy cleanup.
- ♥ Toaster oven. Great for making small meals or reheating certain leftovers.
- ♥ Microwave. Always great for reheating or making quick scrambled eggs.
- ♥ Blender. Can help with pureeing vegetables to sneak into sauces or soups, in addition to making great smoothies.
- ♥ Digital kitchen scale. Helps make it easy to avoid "portion distortion."
- ♥ Food processor. Makes it a breeze to cut up vegetables.
- ♥ Mandoline or V-Slicer. Even faster cut up veggies.
- ♥ Instant-read digital thermometers. Tell you when your meat is cooked correctly, and when your leftovers are heated enough (165°).
- ♥ Great super sharp knives, not serrated. Make cutting up vegetables easier. Thinner blades are easier to push through larger vegetables.

Cookbooks, Recipes

Some cookbooks that are supportive of the DASH diet include the following:

Quick and Easy

For the person who likes convenience and needs ideas that are fast, but still wonderful.

Cooking Light's 5 Ingredient, 15 Minute Cookbook by Anne Chappell Cain, Oxford House, 1999.

Cooking Light One-Dish Meals Cookbook by Susan McIntosh, Oxford House.

Lickety Split Meals by Zonya Foco, ZHI Publishing, 1998.

Quick & Healthy, Low-Fat, Carb Conscious Cooking, by Brenda J. Ponichtera, ScaleDown Publishing, Inc., 2004

Absolute Must-have

Better Homes and Garden New Cook Book, 12th Edition, Meredith Books, 2002. (Older versions of this cookbook are also fabulous.)

For the Serious Cook

Anything by Julia Child, including, *The Way to Cook*, Julia Child, Knopf, 1989.

Roasting. A Simple Art, Barbara Kafka, William Morrow and Company, Inc. 1995.

Le Cordon Bleu Complete Cooking Techniques, Jeni Wright & Eric Treuille, Cassell PLC, 1996.

Websites for DASH-friendly recipes:

FIND RECIPES FOR LEAN BEEF AND PORK
http://www.beefitswhatsfordinner.com

http://www.otherwhitemeat.com

LOW-FAT AND NONFAT DAIRY RECIPES
http://nationaldairycouncil.com

http://www.ilovecheese.com/recipes.asp

ADD MORE FRUITS AND VEGETABLES TO YOUR DIET
http://www.fruitsandveggiesmorematters.org/?page_id=5

INCLUDE NUTS, BEANS, AND SOY

http://www.almondboard.com/recipes/

http://www.michiganbean.org/recipes

http://www.pea-lentil.com/cookbook.htm

http://www.walnuts.org/walnuts/index.cfm/all-recipes/

http://www.soyconnection.com

http://www.soyfoods.com/recipes/

For more Websites and updates on the above sites, see
http://dashdiet.org/dash_diet_recipe_links.asp

DASHboard

1. Stock up on DASH foods.
2. Refrigerator: 2% or low-fat cheeses, fresh veggies from the salad bar, bagged cut-up vegetables, fresh fruit, lean meats, fish.
3. Freezer: frozen vegetables, frozen fruit, 95% extra-lean ground sirloin and patties, boneless and skinless chicken breasts, diced peppers and onions.
4. Cupboards: seasonings, canned no-salt beans, no added salt tomato products, including sauce, diced and whole tomatoes. Sugar substitutes.
5. Equipment: countertop grill, food processor, great knives, microwave, blender, instant-read thermometer.
6. Great cookbooks provide lots of ideas for your DASH diet meals.
7. More recipes can be found at the Websites listed at the end of this chapter.

Tracking my Personal DASH Diet Action Plan

Items I plan to add to my kitchen include:_____

_____

_____

_____

_____

CHAPTER 16

FABULOUS RECIPES FOR THE DASH TO SUCCESS

GROUND BEEF (EXTRA-LEAN) RECIPES

"PILE IT ON!" CHILI

So named because it tastes great and it piles on vegetables. This chili is very low in calories because of all the vegetables. You will get full before you can overdo this great tasting chili. Top with shredded light cheese and baked tortilla strips, if desired.

    1 pound ground sirloin, 95% extra-lean
    ½ bag frozen onion and sliced peppers combo
    2 - 3 garlic cloves, minced or squeezed through a garlic press
    1 14½-oz. can diced tomatoes, no added salt
    1 15-oz. can tomato sauce, no added salt
    1 15½-oz. can kidney beans
    1 can black beans
    2 tablespoons chili powder

2 tablespoons paprika
½ bag frozen mixed broccoli, cauliflower, and carrots
1 cup frozen corn

Heat a large nonstick skillet over medium-high heat. Add ground beef (you can substitute ground turkey breast, if desired), cook 3 minutes, turn down heat to medium. Add peppers, onions, and garlic. (High temperatures make garlic turn bitter and brown.) Continue cooking about 5 more minutes, or until thoroughly browned and onions are soft.

Add tomatoes, beans and seasonings. Mix well; allow to simmer about 5 minutes. Then add mixed vegetables and corn.

Simmer 30 - 60 minutes. If the chili starts getting really thick, you could add water or more tomato sauce.

Yield: Twelve 1-cup servings. Nutrition DASHboard: 204 calories, 13 g protein, 24 g carbohydrates, 7 g fat, 26 mg cholesterol, 7 g fiber, 379 mg sodium, 583 mg potassium.

Alternatives: If you prefer, you can use diced fresh onions, and red, green, and yellow pepper strips. You can add any other vegetables that you think would be interesting. Friends from Texas tell me that sweet potato chunks are wonderful in chili.

BAKED TORTILLA STRIPS

Cut 2 corn tortillas into ½-inch strips. Place on tray in oven or toaster oven. Heat at 400° for 5 minutes, or until lightly browned. Use to garnish the chili.

Sloppy Joes

1 pound extra-lean ground beef, 95% lean
1 cup chopped onions, fresh or frozen
1 cup chopped green peppers, fresh or frozen
2 garlic cloves, minced or squeezed through a garlic press
1 15-oz. can red tomato sauce, no salt added
2 tablespoons red wine vinegar
1 teaspoon paprika
2 teaspoons Worcestershire sauce
½ teaspoon chili powder
½ teaspoon black pepper
dash (or more) hot pepper sauce or cayenne pepper

Heat a large nonstick skillet over medium-high heat. Add ground beef, cook 3 minutes, turn down heat to medium. Add peppers, onions, and garlic. (High temperatures make garlic turn bitter, so don't add too early.) Continue cooking 5 or more minutes, or until thoroughly browned.

Add tomato sauce and all other ingredients. Reduce heat and simmer 10 - 15 minutes.

Yield: 5 servings. Nutrition DASHboard: 224 calories, 27 g protein, 13 g carbohydrates, 7 g fat, 76 mg cholesterol, 2 g fiber, 114 mg sodium, 798 mg potassium.

Extra-Lean Meaty Spaghetti Sauce

1 pound extra-lean ground beef, 95% lean
2 garlic cloves, minced or squeezed through garlic press
½ cup chopped onions, fresh or frozen
1 15-oz. can tomato sauce, no salt added
1 14½-oz. can diced tomatoes, no salt added
1 teaspoon Italian seasoning
1 teaspoon dried basil

Heat a large nonstick skillet over medium-high heat. Add ground beef, cook 3 minutes, turn down heat to medium. Add onions and garlic. Continue cooking about 5 more minutes, or until thoroughly browned. (High temperatures make garlic turn bitter so don't add too early.)

Add diced tomatoes and tomato sauce. Simmer 10 - 15 minutes. Add seasonings in last few minutes of cooking.

Yield: 6 servings. Nutrition DASHboard: 184 calories, 24 g protein, 8 g carbohydrates, 6 g fat, 67 mg cholesterol, 2 g fiber, 105 mg sodium, 733 mg potassium.

Extra-Lean Beef Taco Filling

1 pound extra lean ground sirloin, 95% lean
½ bottle mild or medium taco sauce
1 cup diced onions, fresh or frozen
1 cup diced green peppers, fresh or frozen

Heat a large nonstick skillet over medium-high heat. Add ground beef, cook 3 minutes, turn down heat to medium. Add onions and peppers. Continue cooking 5 or more minutes, or until thoroughly browned.

Add taco sauce, reduce heat and simmer 5 - 10 minutes.

Yield: 4 servings (enough for 3 medium-sized tacos for each serving). Nutrition DASHboard: 140 calories, 17 g protein, 7 g carbohydrates, 4 g fat, 48 mg cholesterol, 1 g fiber, 164 mg sodium, 344 mg potassium.

CHICKEN RECIPES

LOW-SODIUM CHICKEN PICCATA

1 pound chicken breasts, boneless, skinless (4 half-breasts)
½ cup yellow cornmeal
1 teaspoon lemon-pepper seasoning mix
1 cup low-sodium chicken broth
1 tablespoon olive oil
2 tablespoons lemon juice
2 tablespoons butter

Preheat chicken broth over medium heat.

Place each chicken breast half on a sheet of plastic wrap. Sprinkle with water, then place another sheet of plastic wrap on top. (The water keeps the wrap from sticking together and makes it easier to peel apart.) Pound chicken to about ¼ inch thickness using a mallet or rolling pin.

Mix cornmeal and pepper on a plate or pie pan. Drag chicken through cornmeal mix, coating both sides well. (Note: if you want to lower the calories or carb content, you can omit this step and just sprinkle the lemon-pepper seasonings on the chicken.)

Heat oil in a large nonstick skillet over medium-high heat. (If the oil is smoking the temperature is too high.) Add chicken and cook 4 minutes on each side or until browned. Remove chicken from pan, place on plate with cover (pot lid or bowl), to keep warm.

Add lemon juice and hot chicken broth to skillet, scraping pan to loosen browned bits. Reduce heat to medium, stir in butter. Return chicken to pan, cook 3 minutes or until done (internal temperature 165°F). Remove from heat, serve immediately.

Yield: 4 servings. Nutrition DASHboard: 287 calories, 28 g protein, 20 g carbohydrate, 12 g fat, 82 mg cholesterol, 94 mg sodium, 299 mg potassium.

Recipe adapted from *Sara Moulton Cooks at Home*.

CARIBBEAN CHICKEN

1 pound chicken breasts, boneless, skinless (4 half-breasts)
1 teaspoon salt
dash pepper
dash onion powder
dash garlic powder
dash cayenne pepper
dash paprika
1 tablespoon vegetable oil
1 13¼-oz. can pineapple chunks
1 teaspoon ginger
2 oranges, one for juice and peel, one for peeled orange slices
¼ cup honey
2 teaspoons flour
2 tablespoons water
1 orange, peeled and sliced

Season chicken with salt, pepper, onion powder, garlic powder, paprika, and cayenne pepper. Sauté in hot oil until well browned on all sides. Drain excess fat.

Drain pineapple, and reserve juice for sauce. Combine pineapple juice, ginger, 2 teaspoons orange peel, a cup orange juice (squeezed from orange) and honey. Pour over chicken. Cover and simmer 40 minutes or until tender.

Remove chicken to a warm serving platter.

Mix flour and water together until smooth. Stir into pan drippings, and heat to boiling while stirring. Add pineapple chunks and orange slices from second orange (remove peel). Heat just until fruit is warm, serve over chicken.

Yield: 6 servings. Nutrition DASHboard: 295 calories, 27 g protein, 36 g carbohydrates, 5 g fat, 66 mg cholesterol, 2 mg fiber, 83 mg sodium, 371 mg potassium.

CHICKEN CACCIATORE

1½ pounds boneless, skinless chicken breasts
1 14½-oz. can stewed tomatoes, no added salt
1 package frozen sliced onion and pepper combo
1 teaspoon Italian herb seasoning
1 15-oz. can tomato sauce, no added salt
¼ teaspoon red pepper flakes

Spray a large saucepan with non-stick coating. Add chicken and remaining ingredients.

Cover and simmer, stirring occasionally, for 25-35 minutes.

Yield: 4 servings. Nutrition DASHboard 185 calories, 28 g protein, 14 g carbohydrate, 2 g fat, 66 mg cholesterol, 3 g fiber, 122 mg sodium, 808 mg potassium.

Alternatively, this recipe could be prepared in a slow cooker. If you are having potatoes with the meal, slice them, and place them underneath the chicken before cooking.

POLLO ALLA GRIGLIO

This is grilled chicken, pan-finished with lemon sauce, placed on top of baby greens, with roasted potatoes. You could also substitute chicken piccata for the grilled chicken.

1 pound chicken breast, skinless boneless
1 tablespoon olive oil
1 garlic clove
1 cup low-sodium chicken broth
2 tablespoons lemon juice
¼ teaspoon ground black pepper
2 tablespoons butter
½ teaspoon poultry seasoning
4 medium red potatoes, quartered
1 tablespoon olive oil
nonstick cooking spray
baby greens
20 grape tomatoes

Preheat oven to 400°. Quarter potatoes, place in small roasting pan, drizzle with olive oil or spray with nonstick cooking spray. Roast in 400° oven for 30 minutes.

Heat chicken broth over medium heat.

Rub chicken breasts with cut garlic clove, and sprinkle with mixed sage and rosemary. Spray chicken with nonstick cooking spray and place on hot grill. Cook 4 minutes on each side, or until browned. Place grilled chicken on plate and cover with pot lid or aluminum foil.

Heat 1 tablespoon olive oil in large, nonstick skillet over medium heat. Add warm chicken broth, lemon juice, ground pepper, and butter. Place grilled chicken and roasted potatoes in sauce, and heat 3 - 4 minutes, turning to coat with sauce.

Place on top of baby greens and grape tomatoes.

Yield: 4 servings. Nutrition DASHboard: 349 calories, 30 g protein, 23 g carbohydrate, 15 g fat, 83 mg cholesterol, 152 mg sodium, 866 mg potassium.

Roasted Chicken with Potatoes, Carrots, and Brussels Sprouts

1 whole chicken, about 5 pounds
4 medium potatoes, with skin, cut into large chunks
2 cups Brussels sprouts
2 cups carrots, sliced into 1" sections
1 tablespoon olive oil
1 teaspoon poultry seasoning

Preheat oven to 350°F. Place washed and dried chicken in roasting pan. Dust with poultry seasoning, inside and out.

Place cut-up potatoes, sliced carrots, and Brussels sprouts around chicken, drizzle with olive oil. Add 1 cup water to bottom of pan (or white wine or low-sodium chicken broth).

Roast in 350° oven for 60 minutes.

Yield: 4 servings. Nutrition DASHboard: 319 calories, 32 g protein, 42 g carbohydrates, 3 g fat, 66 mg cholesterol, 7 g fiber, 142 mg sodium, 1465 mg potassium.

Alternately you could use a frozen mixture of carrots, cauliflower, and broccoli.

Pepper-Slaw Chicken Stir-Fry

1 pound boneless, skinless chicken breasts, cut into
   ½" x 2" strips
½ bag broccoli slaw
½ bag frozen onion and pepper mixture (or for less soft
   texture, use sliced fresh onions and red, orange, yellow
   and green peppers)
low-sodium stir-fry sauce
2 tablespoons peanut oil or canola oil

Heat a large skillet over medium-high heat. Add peanut (or canola) oil.

When oil is hot (but not smoking), add ½ of chicken strips to oil, and sauté 1 -2 minutes, stirring with wooden spatula until cooked on all sides.

Remove chicken, place on warm plate, repeat with rest of chicken. Cover plate with pot lid or aluminum foil to keep warm.

Add pepper and onion mixture to pan. Stir-fry 3 - 4 minutes. (Watch out for splatters from the moisture if you use frozen vegetables.) Add broccoli slaw, and sauté until tender.

Add ¼ cup stir-fry sauce, and place chicken back into pan. Stir well to reheat chicken and to mix sauce.

Yield: 4 (2-cup) servings. Nutrition DASHboard: 235 calories, 29 g protein, 10 g carbohydrates, 9 g fat, 66 mg cholesterol, 3 g fiber, 184 g sodium, 610 mg potassium.

Alternate recipe: Chinese Vegetable Stir-Fry. Same basic recipe as above, substituting for the vegetables: chopped bok choi, water chestnuts, sliced mushrooms, and bean sprouts. You can find frozen stir-fry mixtures that also work well. Be careful of splatters when adding frozen vegetables to hot oil.

PORK RECIPES

Peach-Mustard Glazed Pork Chops

4 4-oz. boneless pork loin chops, ¾ inch thick (trim
  all visible fat)
1 16-oz. can peach slices in extra light syrup, undrained
2 tablespoons peach preserves
2 tablespoons Dijon mustard
1 teaspoon Worcestershire sauce
1 teaspoon black pepper

Combine peaches, preserves, mustard, and Worcestershire sauce in medium bowl.

Heat large nonstick skillet over medium-high heat until hot.

Season chops with pepper. Add chops to skillet; brown on both sides.

Add peach mixture to skillet; reduce heat to low. Cover; cook 5 minutes. Serve pork chops topped with peach mixture. Garnish with fresh raspberries, if desired.

Yield: 4 servings. Nutrition DASHboard: 236 calories, 22 g protein, 15 g carbohydrate, 10 g fat, 73 mg cholesterol, 96 mg sodium, 458 mg potassium.

Recipe from National Pork Producers Council.

BEAN RECIPES

Beans are not a common part of the typical American diet. The following recipes were developed or modified by my students at the University of Illinois at Chicago in an introductory foods class. All of the recipes were favorites. Since college students are notoriously picky, you can be sure that these very appetizing recipes will help you expand your own repertoire of bean dishes.

RICE WITH BLACK-EYED PEAS & TOMATOES

1 tablespoon olive oil
1 large onion, peeled and finely chopped
1 garlic clove, peeled and finely chopped or squeezed
   through a garlic press
1 ½ cups long-grain white rice
1 16-oz. can black-eyed peas, undrained
1 28-oz. can diced tomatoes, drained
1½ tablespoons chili powder
½ teaspoon cumin
1 teaspoon crushed dried oregano
¼ teaspoon cayenne pepper
3 cups water
dash salt, pepper

Add olive oil to nonstick skillet, over medium heat.

When oil is hot, add onion and sauté until translucent, about 5 minutes. Reduce the heat to prevent browning, and add garlic and continue to sauté until lightly browned. (Do not cook the garlic at too high a heat or allow to get dark, since it will turn bitter.)

Put the sautéed onions and garlic into a large pot, add the remaining ingredients, and bring to a boil over medium-high heat, stirring occasionally.

Reduce the heat and simmer, partially covered, until the rice is tender, about 30 minutes, stirring occasionally to ensure that everything is evenly distributed.

Season with pepper to taste.

Yield: 8 (1-cup) servings. Nutrition DASHboard: 230 calories, 5 g protein, 47 g carbohydrates, 2 g fat, 6 g fiber, 61 mg sodium, 568 mg potassium.

LENTIL CONFETTI SALAD

1 cup lentils, rinsed
3 cups water
1 cup white rice, cooked and warm
½ cup light Italian dressing
1 large tomato, seeded and diced
½ cup finely diced red onion
½ cup celery, chopped
¼ cup pimento stuffed olives, sliced
¼ cup sweet green pepper, medium diced
1 tablespoon fresh parsley, chopped

In a saucepan, pour water over lentils, bring to a boil, and simmer 20 minutes or until lentils are tender.

Separately, cook rice per package directions. *Note: this recipe calls for 1 cup of cooked rice.*

Combine drained lentils with rice and all vegetables.

Toss lightly with dressing.

Yield: 8 servings. Nutrition DASHboard: 131 calories, 8 g protein, 22 g carbohydrates, 2 g fat, 8 g fiber, 99 g sodium, 321 mg potassium.

Recipe adapted from USA Dry Pea & Lentil Council

BLACK BEANS WITH TOMATOES AND CILANTRO*

This is a wonderful, healthy dip for baked corn tortillas (whole grain) or for cut up pepper strips.

1 15-oz. can black beans, drained and rinsed
1 ½ tablespoon peanut or corn oil
1 medium onion, chopped
1 teaspoon garlic, chopped
1 14½-oz. can diced tomatoes, drained
½ teaspoon Tabasco sauce
½ teaspoon salt
2 tablespoons fresh cilantro, chopped

Heat oil in a small skillet over medium high-heat; add the onions and garlic. Sauté, stirring until onion is almost translucent but still firm, about 2 minutes. Add tomatoes and cook, Stirring frequently, for 2 minutes more.

Add black beans, Tabasco, and salt. Stir to combine. Cover skillet. Cook until beans are heated through about 2 minutes.

Remove from heat. Stir in 1 tablespoon of cilantro. Transfer to serving dish and sprinkle with remaining cilantro. Serve immediately.

Yield: 8 (½-cup) servings. Nutrition DASHboard: 110 calories, 5 g protein, 17 g carbohydrates, 3 g fat, 6 g fiber, 23 mg sodium, 333 mg potassium.

PASTA E FAGIOLI ALLA VENEZIA*

1 15-oz. can kidney beans
¼ cup olive oil
1 cup onion, chopped coarse
1 cup carrot, chopped coarse
1 celery stalk with leaves, chopped coarse
1 tablespoon garlic, chopped fine
3 tablespoons fresh basil, chopped fine, or 1 teaspoon
  dried basil
1 cup canned Italian plum tomatoes, chopped
1 teaspoon dried rosemary, crushed
¼ teaspoon red pepper flakes
¼ teaspoon dried sage
2 cups low-sodium chicken or vegetable broth, or boiling water
2 cups dried whole grain pasta

Heat oil in large heavy saucepan over medium-high heat. Add onions and sauté until they begin to turn golden. Add carrot, celery, and garlic. Cook for a few minutes more, stirring occasionally.

Add beans, tomatoes, rosemary, sage, red pepper flakes, and 1 cup boiling liquid. Turn heat to high and bring to boil. Reduce heat to simmer. Cook covered, until beans are tender, about 15 minutes.

Transfer about 2 ladles of beans and their liquid to food processor, blender, or food mill. Process to a thick puree and stir back into soup.

About 15 minutes before serving, bring soup to a boil and add pasta and the remaining cup of broth. Stir occasionally, until pasta is cooked al dente, about 8 to 10 minutes.

Remove from heat and stir in pepper to taste.

Ladle into soup bowls and sprinkle each serving with Parmesan cheese.

Yield: 6 servings. Nutrition DASHboard: 167 calories, 8 g protein, 33 g carbohydrates, 1.5 g fat, 7 g fiber, 498 mg sodium, 613 mg potassium.

* Recipes adapted from Michigan Bean Commission

MISCELLANEOUS RECIPES

SOUTHWESTERN EGG WHITE OMELET

½ cup egg substitutes or 4 egg whites
¼ cup diced red bell pepper
1 tablespoon diced jalapeño peppers (if desired)
¼ cup diced onions

Heat nonstick omelet pan or small skillet, over medium heat. Spray with nonstick cooking spray. Sauté peppers and onions until slightly soft.

Pour ½ cup egg substitute or egg whites over onion and pepper mixture. Gently lift sides of omelet, as egg begins to set, to allow uncooked egg to slide underneath and firm up. Repeat until top of omelet is relatively set. Flip once. Allow to cook for a few seconds, then fold over, and slip onto plate.

Yield: 1 serving. Nutrition DASHboard: 90 calories, 13 g protein, 9 g carbohydrates, 0 g fat, 0 mg cholesterol, 2 g fiber, 232 mg sodium, 329 mg potassium.

Alternately, you could use ¼ cup diced tomato, ¼ cup green peppers, and a few sliced mushrooms.

PARMESAN ROASTED RED POTATOES

1 pound new (small) red potatoes
½ cup freshly grated Parmesan cheese
non-stick cooking spray
1 teaspoon dried oregano
1 teaspoon dried basil

Preheat oven to 400°F. In small roasting pan place red potatoes. Spray with nonstick cooking spray. Sprinkle with Parmesan cheese, oregano, and basil. Cook about 40 minutes, or until tender.

Yield: 4 servings. Nutrition DASHboard: 164 calories, 6 g protein, 21 g carbohydrates, 1 g fat, 9 mg cholesterol, 2 g fiber, 159 mg sodium, 493 mg potassium.

LOW-FAT, LOW- SALT TUNA SALAD

1 6-oz. can very low-sodium tuna
2 tablespoons low-fat mayonnaise
¼ cup diced celery
¼ cup diced red peppers
dash ground black pepper

Mix all ingredients together. If you want more color and crunch, you could also add some grated carrots. A diced egg could add some more protein and additional creaminess (although it would significantly increase the cholesterol).

Yield: 2 servings. Nutrition DASHboard: 142 calories, 21 g protein, 1.5 g carbohydrate, 6 g fat, 50 mg cholesterol, 267 mg sodium, 205 mg potassium.

CHICKEN WALDORF SALAD

1 6-oz. can chicken meat
¼ cup diced celery
¼ cup diced apple
2 tablespoons coarsely chopped walnuts
¼ cup light mayonnaise
1 teaspoon lemon juice

Toss chicken, celery, apples, and nuts together lightly. Chill.

Mix salad dressing and lemon juice. Gently stir into chicken mixture. Chill.

Yield: 4 (½-cup) servings. Nutrition DASHboard: 137 calories, 13 g protein, 4 g carbohydrates, 8 g fat, 41 mg cholesterol, 114 mg sodium, 160 mg potassium.

Alternately, for Tuna Waldorf Salad, substitute a can of low-sodium tuna for the chicken.

ITALIAN COLESLAW

1¼ cup shredded cabbage
1/3 cup shredded carrots
1/3 cup green or red bell pepper, sliced
2 tablespoons sliced red onions
2 tablespoons olive oil
3 tablespoons red wine vinegar
¼ teaspoon celery seeds

Mix all ingredients. Chill.

Yield: 6 (½-cup) servings. Nutrition DASHboard: 63 calories, 7 g carbo-hydrates, 4 g fat, 1 g fiber, 16 mg sodium, 153 mg potassium.

HALIBUT IN BALSAMIC REDUCTION

1 pound halibut
1 teaspoon olive oil
1 shallot, minced
1/3 cup balsamic vinegar
½ cup chicken broth, warm

Preheat oven to 450°F. Cut halibut into 4 pieces. Place halibut on baking sheet that has been sprayed with nonstick cooking spray, spray again. Bake in oven 6 - 8 minutes, depending on thickness.

Heat chicken broth for 1 minute in microwave on high.

In small skillet or sauté pan, over medium heat, heat 1 tablespoon olive oil. Add minced shallot; cook until translucent and soft. Add balsamic vinegar and warm chicken broth. Continue to cook over medium-high heat until volume is reduced by half.

SMASHED RED POTATOES

2 pounds red potatoes, cut into large chunks
4 - 8 oz. skim milk (warm)
¼ teaspoon ground black pepper
1 tablespoon butter, soft or melted

Cut potatoes (do not peel) into large chunks, 1 ½ - 2". Cook 20-25 min-utes in boiling water until very tender. When the potatoes are done, drain, and put back in pan to allow excess moisture to evaporate. Add butter, pepper, and skim milk according to the desired consistency. Mash gently, leaving skins relatively intact.

Yield: 6 servings. Nutrition DASHboard: 145 calories, 4 g protein, 28 g carbohydrate, 2 g fat, 6 mg cholesterol, 2 g fiber, 31 mg sodium, 652 mg potassium.

OVEN POTATO FRIES

4 medium baking potatoes (about 1½ - 2 pounds)
2 teaspoons salt-free seasoning mix (or ½ teaspoon pepper,
  1 teaspoon paprika, ½ teaspoon onion powder,
  ½ teaspoon garlic powder)
1 tablespoon vegetable oil
nonstick cooking spray

Preheat oven to 450°F.

Slice potatoes into wedges, with a maximum width of ½ inch. Place potato slices, oil, and seasonings into a plastic zipper bag. Shake well to distribute seasonings on potato surfaces.

Spray baking sheet with nonstick cooking spray. Arrange potato slices on baking sheet. (To minimize clean up, you can line baking sheet first with aluminum foil.)

Bake at 450°F for 30 - 35 minutes, or until golden brown.

Yield: 6 servings. Nutrition DASHboard: 147 calories, 3.5 g protein, 29 g carbohydrates, 2.5 g fat, 0 mg cholesterol, 3 g fiber, 14 mg sodium, 732 mg potassium.

CALORIES AND FAT FOR MEAT AND POULTRY

Calories and Fat for 3-oz. Cooked Lean Beef

	Calories	Fat g	Saturated fat g	Cholesterol mg
Top round roast, broiled	153	4.2	1.4	71
Eye-Round, roasted	143	4.2	1.5	59
Shoulder pot roast, roasted	136	4.7	1.6	54
Round tip roast, roasted	147	5.7	1.8	60
Shoulder steak, braised	161	6.0	1.9	80
Top sirloin steak, broiled	166	6.1	2.4	76
Bottom round, roasted	161	6.3	2.1	66
Top loin steak, broiled	176	8.0	3.1	65
Tenderloin steak, broiled	175	8.1	3.0	71
T-bone steak, broiled	172	8.2	3.0	48
Tri-tip roast, roasted	177	8.2	3.0	70
NY strip steak, broiled				
Ground beef, 95% lean, pan-broiled	139	5.0	2.2	65
Ground beef, 90% lean, pan-broiled	173	9.1	3.7	70
Ground beef, 85% lean, pan-broiled	197	11.9	4.7	73

Calories and Fat for 3-oz. Cooked Lean Pork

	Calories	Fat g	Saturated fat g	Cholesterol mg
Pork tenderloin, roasted	140	4	1	65
Pork top loin roast, roasted	170	6	2	65
Pork top loin chop, broiled	170	7	2	70
Pork loin center chop, broiled	170	7	3	70
Pork sirloin roast, roasted	180	9	3	75
Ham, lean, roasted	145	5.5	1.8	53

Calories and Fat for 3-oz. Cooked Lean Poultry

	Calories	Fat g	Saturated fat g	Cholesterol mg
Chicken breast, with skin, roasted	167	6.6	1.9	71
Chicken breast, skinless, roasted	140	3.0	0.9	72
Chicken thigh, with skin, roasted	210	13.2	3.7	79
Chicken thigh, skinless, roasted	178	9.2	2.6	81
Turkey breast, skinless, roasted	115	0.6	0.2	71
Turkey whole, with skin, roasted	146	4.9	1.4	89
Ground turkey, cooked	200	11.2	2.9	87
Ground turkey breast, cooked	98	3.8	1.0	44

Calories and Fat for 3-oz. Cooked Fish and Seafood

	Calories	Fat g	Saturated fats g	Cholesterol mg
Blue crab	100	1	0	90
Catfish	140	9	2	50
Clams (about 12 small)	100	1.5	0	55
Cod	90	0.5	0	45
Flounder/sole	100	1.5	0.5	60
Haddock	100	1	0	80
Halibut	110	2	0	35
Lobster	80	0	0	60
Mackerel	210	13	1.5	60
Ocean perch	110	2	0	50
Orange roughy	80	1	0	20
Oysters, about 12 medium	100	3.5	1	115
Pollock	90	1	0	80
Rainbow trout	140	6	2	60
Rockfish	100	2	0	40
Salmon, Atlantic/Coho	160	7	1	50
Salmon, Chum/Pink	130	4	1	70
Salmon, Sockeye	180	9	1.5	75
Scallops, 6 large, 14 small	120	1	0	55
Shrimp	80	1	0	165
Swordfish	130	4.5	1	40
Tuna, canned in water	116	0.8	0.2	30
White fish	172	7.5	1.2	77

OMEGA-3 FATTY ACID CONTENT FOR FISH AND SEAFOOD

Food Item	EPA (grams)	DHA (grams)
Cod liver oil (1 tablespoon)	1.0	1.5
Mackerel (3.5 ounces)	0.9	1.4
Salmon (3.5 ounces)	0.8	0.6
Herring (3.5 ounces)	0.7	0.9
Anchovy (3.5 ounces)	0.5	0.9
Tuna (3.5 ounces)	0.3	0.9
Blue fish (3.5 ounces)	0.2	0.5
Swordfish (3.5 ounces)	0.1	0.5

EPA = eicosapentaenoic acid
DHA = docosahexenoic acid

SERVING SIZES

GRAINS

The serving sizes are designed to be about 1 ounce dry weight and about 80 calories. Watch out for cereal serving sizes that can range from ¼ cup to 1½ cups.

1 slice bread
½ cup cooked pasta, rice, cereal, corn
1 oz. dry cereal
¼ bagel
½ English muffin or hamburger or hot dog bun
2 cups popcorn
2 small cookies

FRUITS

6 oz. juice
medium fruit
¼ cup dried fruit
½ cup canned fruit
1 cup large diced raw fruit

VEGETABLES

½ cup cooked vegetables
1 cup leafy greens
6 oz. vegetable juice

DAIRY

8 oz. skim or low-fat milk
8 oz. low-fat/fat-free yogurt
1 oz. reduced-fat cheese
½ cup fat-free or low-fat cottage cheese

BEANS, NUTS, SEEDS

¼ cup beans
¼ cup or 1 oz. nuts, seeds

LEAN MEAT, FISH, POULTRY, EGGS

3 oz. is about the size of a deck of cards or the palm of a woman's hand

1 egg = 1 oz.
2 egg whites = 1 oz.

FATS, FATTY SAUCES

1 tablespoon salad dressing
1 teaspoon butter, oil

INDEX

ACKNOWLEDGMENTS

Many people have helped and supported me while I wrote this book. First, I received research support and ideas for menu plans from two dietetic interns from the University of Illinois at Chicago, Andrea Denk and Susan Nordmark. Heidi Hartman, a dietetic intern from the University of Delaware performed much of the work in developing the analysis of the menu plans.

Susan Moores provided editing support on early drafts of several chapters of the book.

I was introduced to the DASH Diet by Shiriki Kumanyika, PhD, RD, who has extensive research background in research and management of hypertension, and was involved in the initial development of the DASH diet concept. Shiriki was also my master's thesis advisor.

I also had the pleasure of arranging for Marlene Most, PhD, RD, to speak at an Illinois Dietetic Association meeting. She was a key developer of the DASH Diet, one of the lead researchers, and is published frequently on the DASH Diet research.

My clients continue to provide me with the opportunity to learn how better to support dietary behavior change.

I continue to be grateful for the superior education and continuing guidance I have received in this, my second career, from my professors at Dominican University (Judy Beto, PhD, RD, and Betsy Holli, PhD, RD) and at the University of Illinois at Chicago (Bob Reynolds, PhD; Phyllis Bowen, PhD, RD; Noel Chavez, PhD, RD; and Savitri Kamath, PhD, RD).

I also greatly benefited from my students in the introductory foods classes and the nutrition education and counseling classes. They helped me develop recipes, some of which are found in this book, and focus on actions that help people adopt sustainable behavior changes.

My graduate coursework in health behavior and health promotion strengthened my focus on helping people make sustainable behavior changes. My epidemiology coursework reinforced the importance of controlling the epidemics of hypertension, heart disease, type 2 diabetes, and obesity.

And finally, I want to thank my husband, Richard, who has supported me in my endeavors over the five years it took to complete this book. He has been a never ending source of encouragement, support, and love. I am truly grateful to him.

ABOUT THE AUTHOR

Marla Heller has devoted most of her professional career in nutrition to promoting the DASH diet and showing that it can be adopted and sustained by the general public. She is a registered dietitian and holds a master of science in human nutrition and dietetics from the University of Illinois at Chicago (UIC), where she completed course work towards a PhD in behavior sciences and health promotion. Most recently she was employed by the US Department of Health and Human Services. She also has run a private practice in nutrition and dietetics, worked at the Naval Hospital, Great Lakes, providing nutrition counseling for active-duty and retired military personnel and their families, and at the University of Illinois Hospital in the Heart-Lung Transplant Unit and the Cardiac Step-Down Unit. She has been an adjunct clinical instructor in foods and nutrition at UIC, Dominican University, and National-Louis University. She was a faculty member at the Cooking and Hospitality Institute of Chicago, teaching nutrition to student chefs.

In addition to *The DASH Diet Action Plan*, Marla wrote the four-week menu plan for *Win the Weight Game* by Sarah Ferguson, the Duchess of York. She has been a featured nutrition expert for the *Chicago Tribune*, the *Washington Post*, and WGN-AM. She has frequently presented seminars at corporations, schools, health clubs, and athletic facilities and has been a spokesperson for the Greater Midwest affiliate of the American Heart Association.

She is a past president of the Illinois Dietetic Association, and a past president of the North Suburban Dietetic Association. She was awarded the prestigious Emerging Leader Award from the Illinois Dietetic Association.

Marla was diagnosed with high blood pressure in May of 2003. Since that time she has managed to keep her blood pressure in the normal range by following the DASH diet and exercising. Marla lives the program that is featured in this book and the seminars she presents.

Marla lives with her husband, Richard, in Northbrook, Illinois, where she enjoys cooking, gardening, exercising, and writing.